From Baby to Bikini

From Baby to Bikini

Keep Your Midsection Toned
SAFELY
during Pregnancy
and Flatten Your Abdominals
FAST
after You Have Your Baby

GREG WAGGONER

WITH

DOUG STUMPF

WARNER BOOKS

A Time Warner Company

A NOTE FROM THE PUBLISHER: Neither this program nor any other diet/exercise program should be followed with-out first consulting a healthcare professional. If you have any special conditions requiring attention, you should consult with your healthcare professional regularly regarding possible modification of the program contained in this book.

Grateful acknowledgment is given for permission to reprint from the following:

The "Contraindications to Exercise" quoted on p. 10 are reproduced with permission of The American College of Obstetricians and Gynecologists. *Exercise During Pregnancy and the Postpartum Period* (Technical Bulletin No. 189), Washington, D.C. © ACOG, February 1994.

Recipes on pages 124 and 125 are reprinted from *The Low-Carb Cookbook: The Complete Guide to the Healthy Low-Carbohydrate Lifestyle—with Over 250 Delicious Recipes, Everything You Need to Know about Stocking the Pantry, and Sources for the Best Prepared Foods and Ingredients* by Fran McCullough. Copyright 1997 by Frances McCullough. Published by Hyperion.

Copyright © 1999 by Greg Waggoner and Doug Stumpf

All rights reserved.

Warner Books, Inc., 1271 Avenue of the Americas, New York, NY 10020

Visit our Web site at www.warnerbooks.com

 A Time Warner Company

Printed in the United States of America

First Printing: June 1999

10 9 8 7 6 5 4 3

Library of Congress Cataloging-in-Publication Data

Waggoner, Greg.

    From baby to bikini : keep your midsection toned safely during pregnancy and flatten your abdominals fast after you have your baby / Greg Waggoner with Doug Stumpf.

    p. cm.

  ISBN 0-446-67398-6

  1. Exercise for pregnant women—Popular works. 2. Physical fitness for women—Popular works. 3. Prenatal care—Popular works. 4. Postnatal care—Popular works. I. Stumpf, Doug. II. Title.

  RG558.7 .W34 1999

  618.2'4—ddc21   98-37516

                                                                        CIP

Cover design by Elaine Groh

Cover photo by Gaspar Tringle

Book design and text composition by Spinning Egg Design Group

Acknowledgments

I want to express my sincerest gratitude to the following people who helped me with this book: Dr. Phyllis Carr, Dr. Mike Makii, Dr. James Clapp, and RoseMarie Dixon for reading the manuscript and making suggestions; Marlene Nadler and Christine Scarcelli, my colleagues from Equinox, and who prove as models in the photographs that it is possible to be both a mother and in top physical condition; Patrick and Kara Fowler for making available my smallest model; Gaspar Tringle for his fantastic photos and calming influence; Mary Evans, literary agent extraordinaire; Sandra Bark at Warner Books; Doug Stumpf for encouraging me to write this book and for helping turn my ideas into words; my editor, Amy Einhorn, for sharing and shaping my vision and for her incredibly perceptive and meticulous advice and editing; and my parents, for encouraging my interest in health and fitness and for giving me the kind of love and support that enables me to pursue my dreams.

~ Greg Waggoner

Contents

Foreword

There is nothing quite like motherhood and a new baby. Those first few days are filled with such delight, and the early weeks are so sleepless, that you barely notice what has become of your figure. Then one day you step out from the shower (the first free moment you have had in weeks), and you accidentally glance into the mirror. That maternal glow dims as you realize that those pounds you packed on so easily while "eating for two" are no longer bringing joy and smiles into your life. The task of regaining a fit and well-toned body seems impossible, overwhelming. You don't have the time, work looms, the baby is crying, and you desperately need a nap.

Actually, what you need is this book.

This book is special because it brings the knowledge and skill of a personal trainer to your side. Greg Waggoner has enjoyed years of experience and success as a personal trainer for pregnant women and new mothers. His knowledge and common sense make this book a delight to read. It is reassuring to know that the exercises you will be doing have been used by an experienced trainer to help other women remain fit during and after pregnancy. The photographs and easy-to-follow exercise instructions help the reader to embark on a program that encourages a fit pregnancy and an easy recovery.

Greg then turns to the postpartum period. He offers lifestyle advice along with a detailed exercise program. The program is carefully paced, beginning with a routine that, while not overtaxing, is challenging enough to produce the desired results. Seeing early results is encouraging, and over the next weeks of the program the pace increases. Soon the results become more noticeable to you and to those around you.

Because Greg realizes that each woman may be at a different level of conditioning (both during and after pregnancy), he offers suggestions on how to modify each exercise routine for your individual needs. This is one of the key reasons that the program is so successful and why it is so much like having your own trainer. Besides exercises and stretching, the book also provides dietary tips, including some delicious and healthy recipes, that are helpful as you increase your activities or return to work.

As a physician and mother I have read and tried all types of quick fixes and fad exercise programs. Most of them either don't work or are too boring or impossible to incorporate into an already busy life. I wish that *From Baby to Bikini* had been around a few years ago when I gave birth to my children. However, even women who had their babies a few years ago can benefit from this book! The program is easy to follow, fun to do, and, along with great results, will help you develop lifelong fitness and health.

—Renee Garrick, M.D.

Introduction: Why This Book?

Recently I was at a party where I was introduced as a fitness trainer. One man came up and asked me to speak to his wife, who had just had her second child and was worried about getting back into shape. The man brought me over to a woman who was standing by herself and obviously not having a very good time. She seemed clearly depressed as she asked me the usual questions about my work—what kind of clients I had, what sort of exercises I did with them, etc. Suddenly, by accident, she knocked my drink out of my hand. That caused her to break down sobbing. She admitted that she felt terrible about herself, and her body. She was 10 pounds overweight and couldn't fit into any of her old clothes. She believed her husband no longer found her attractive because she was out of shape. She thought her situation was "hopeless." She had given up jogging, which she had once counted on to lift her spirits and keep her weight down. With the new baby and a two-year-old to care for, and a full-time job she would soon go back to, there was no time to work out or prepare special diet meals for herself.

I assured her that she was not alone in her predicament or in the way she felt. I told her about the many new and experienced mothers I've worked with and how they've successfully gotten back into shape within months of delivery. For instance, my client Rhoda came to me when she was 30 years old and had just had her second baby. She was 20 pounds overweight and didn't have the strength in her midsection to do even 1 "crunch" (half sit-up). Within 6 months she was down to her ideal weight, and she was strong enough to do 35 crunches. She would pat her belly and say how tight it felt!

Another client of mine, Sally, a lawyer with 3 children, told me,

I used to think it was a tradeoff—I had to give up exercise and look-
ing good in order to be a good mother. I love my kids—they're the
biggest joy in my life—and I want to spend as much time with them

as possible, which is hard with my job. But now I know I can be a better mother if I stay fit, look good, and feel good about myself. My kids are even proud of the shape I'm in—they brag about it to their friends. They always want to come to the gym with me.

As a fitness trainer in New York City, I work with many different kinds of people with different fitness goals—from competitive athletes to business people to senior citizens—but a large and important group of my clients consists of pregnant women and new mothers. Some were already regular clients before they became pregnant, but many, if not most, have come to me for the first time within a year of having a child. Although few of them are quite so depressed as the woman at the party, most of them share her concerns: their midsections don't feel as toned and firm as they used to; often they gained some weight during pregnancy that stubbornly refuses to come off after childbirth; their bodies have changed and feel different. In one way or another they all ask me the same question: How can I go from having a baby to wearing a bathing suit again and feeling good about it?

I tell them what I told the woman at the party and what I want to tell you now. It's not impossible. It's not even as hard as you think. There *are* ways to find the time, and if you do, you'll find yourself with more energy, not less. Feeling good about your body is a wonderful thing—something no one should give up, ever. The great thing about fitness is that it works for everyone. I've taken people as different as you could possibly imagine and watched their joy as they changed their bodies for the better. Always the results spill over into other areas of their lives: They develop greater self-esteem and confidence. Bodies are not the only thing that change with fitness—so do attitudes and general outlooks. If that isn't enough, and you need one more excuse to get back into shape, here's the best one of all: Feeling better about yourself will make you a better mother!

You'll find it no surprise that the ground-zero concern of new mothers is the abdominal area. It balloons when you are pregnant. After childbirth, the muscles remain stretched but with nothing pushing out against them, they sag. My new-mother clients describe their midsections as "spongy," "mushy," or "abused." Some refer to their condition as "jelly belly."

The other big problem new mothers often encounter is weight gain. Obviously, you are supposed to put on weight during pregnancy. Most of those extra pounds are usually accounted for by the baby, your enlarged uterus and breasts, and fluid. Some of it is fat, however—so-called "maternal stores." Unfortunately this fat does not always automatically disappear after childbirth. Many of my clients tell me they can't get rid of that last 5 or 10 pounds of weight they gained during pregnancy—an especially common complaint after the second or third child. Some women resign themselves to looking "matronly." But there's no reason *you* have to. Believe me, I'm talking from the experience of working successfully with many women. *There's no reason you can't be a mother and still look good and feel good about your body.*

I won't pretend it won't take a bit of work and focus on your part. Being a new mother is demanding, with special requirements. You may feel overextended and tired. Even if your are one of the lucky ones who do not, you can't just launch into a heavy-duty exercise routine and a strict dieting regimen after childbirth. Before beginning any exercise routine, **you must get the permission of your doctor or medical care-giver** (especially if you had any complications during childbirth). You've got to give your body time to recover, which means regaining your strength, endurance, and muscle-tone gradually. In addition, you've got to eat a balanced diet to avoid fatigue (it's not easy, staying up all night with a baby), and, if you are breastfeeding, you must make certain you've eaten enough and enough of the right things so that you and your baby are getting properly nourished.

My new-mother clients tell me over and over the biggest hurdle to overcome is time. There just isn't any.

While I've certainly never had a baby, over the years as I've worked with new mothers I've come to understand the special challenges of this important time in their lives, and I've developed special strategies for helping them cope. Unfortunately, not everyone has access to a personal trainer. I began to wonder what I could do for those women who don't. When I went to the bookstore, I discovered several good overall fitness books for pregnant women, but few for new mothers. Those that do exist are essentially weight-training programs. I do encourage training the whole body (meaning all muscle groups). But the reality is that most new mothers simply can't squeeze in a time-consuming fitness regimen. Traveling to a gym is often out of the question. And, in some cases, I've found that women simply don't enjoy working out with weights. It seems to me that most new mothers want to use the limited time they have for exercise to concentrate on the emergency zone: their midsections.

What I give you here is a book custom-designed for the new mother: an easy-to-use, day-by-day system geared toward returning your midsection to its prepregnancy condition within 24 weeks after childbirth. It takes up as little time as possible—10–20 minutes a day, 3 days a week for the abdominal exercises, and 10–30 minutes a day, 3 days a week of aerobic activity. I also give you diet guidelines and tips developed by fitness-trainer colleagues—some of the healthiest and trimmest people in the world. Wherever possible I try to help you to integrate the system into your busy, new life and show you how to enlist your husband and friends, and even your baby, in your fitness goals. I give you lifestyle hints, so you can use even the tiniest opportunity—like picking up your baby or crossing the street—to help you toward your goal. I try to give you as much variety as possible and to make the whole thing fun. I want this to be an adventure, not a chore.

Time and again I see that my clients who exercise during pregnancy bounce back into top shape after giving birth sooner than those who don't, so I also give you information on how to stay fit *safely* during pregnancy, as well. (If you bought this book after giving birth, you can use those chapters to plan for your next pregnancy and childbirth.)

If you are one of those new mothers who thinks it's impossible to get back into shape, I assure you: If you follow the advice I give in this book, you will be able to change your body dramatically for the better. Sooner than you ever thought possible you'll find yourself making huge improvements and feeling good about the way you look. My goal is to get you on the beach in the bathing suit you want to wear and looking good. I want your husband and your children to feel proud of their active, fit, attractive mom. I want your friends to say to one another, "You won't believe this, but she just had a baby six months ago!" And I'm sure you won't mind if you end up being healthier and feeling better in the process! As I said above, fitness is one of the few things in life that works for *everyone*.

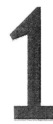

ANATOMY BASICS

Before we get down to the exercises and the "System," let's look at the muscles of the midsection, how they work, and how they are strengthened and made firmer. Some of the terms here are technical and at first some of the concepts might seem like something only a doctor or an exercise professional needs to know, but I think you'll find it well worth the effort to read this chapter. Understanding how your muscles work to make your body move will help you do the exercises correctly—and you need to do an exercise with proper form in order to get the full benefits.

Replacing Fat with Muscle

People have many misconceptions about what muscles are and what they can do. My clients often ask me, "How can I turn my fat into muscle?" Good luck, I tell them. Muscle tissue is completely different from fat tissue—turning it into fat would be as ridiculous as turning an arm into a leg. Fat tissue is where the body stores fat—extra energy or calories. Muscle tissue is made up of protein, and it enables the body to move. *Every* body movement is caused by muscle tissue.

You cannot turn fat tissue into muscle tissue or vice versa. (Some people fear that if they build muscle and then stop working out, it will turn into fat. This is totally irrational.) What you can do is lose fat tissue through diet and aerobic exercise, and strengthen and build muscle tissue through so-called "resistance training," in which you make the muscle work against a resisting force.

How Muscles Work and How Exercise Makes Them Stronger

The only things a muscle can do are contract (shorten) and relax (lengthen.) It seems almost too simple, doesn't it? But this is how your body is able to make—through muscles contracting and relaxing—every movement, from involuntary ones, such as breathing and your heart beating, to voluntary ones, such as walking or picking up a baby.

Every muscle in your body is attached at each end to a bone, a tendon, or another muscle. One end is called the "origin," the other is called the "insertion." This sounds technical, but stay with me. The origin is the most stable attachment of the muscle, meaning when the muscle contracts there is little movement at that end. The insertion—at the other end—is where the most movement occurs. You can do an abdominal crunch because of the main abdominal muscle (the "rectus abdominis"), whose origin is on the top of your pubic bone and whose insertion is just below your breastbone. Notice when you do a crunch, the area of the origin moves very little; most of the movement is at the insertion of the muscle.

Muscles are highly adaptable. For one thing they are elastic. This means they can stretch like a rubber band and snap back—although not instantly; they must adapt over time. As your baby grows inside you, the muscles of the abdominal area stretch to accommodate her increasing size. After you deliver, the muscles gradually return to their normal state—*a process you can accelerate and accentuate through exercise.*

Muscles also adapt to the demands placed upon them by resistance training, that is, they get stronger when they are challenged regularly by work. Your brain and your muscles work together in a system called the "neuromuscular pathway"—to put it simply, your brain tells your muscles to get going! This is how it works: Muscles are made up of individual fibers. As I said above, the only things these fibers can do are contract and relax. When you want to make any movement, your brain sends an electrical impulse down the spinal cord and through the proper nerves to whichever muscles the brain needs to cause the desired movement. The signal from the brain fires the muscle and it contracts, causing its origin and insertion to move toward each other—in the case of the rectus abdominis, the pelvis and the rib cage move toward each other.

Amazingly, your brain calls upon only the exact number of fibers needed in order to accomplish a given, desired movement. Say you bend down to pick up your baby, your brain recruits the exact muscle force needed for you to stand up at the pace you choose. If it couldn't do that, you would jump up in the air every time you stood up. When you have to lift a heavier object, the brain sends the message to more muscle fibers. When these fibers are recruited on a regular basis they grow firmer and stronger. In this way the muscles are more efficiently able to complete the tasks asked of them by the brain. This is how resistance training on a regular basis works to make you more toned and shapely.

The Abdominal Muscles

In this book we are interested mainly in the muscles that make up the abdominal wall. Your abdomen is not the same thing as your stomach. Your stomach is an organ in the digestive system, not a muscle used for movement in the body. As I said previously, the main muscle of the abdominal wall is called the rectus abdominis, which runs down the center of your abdomen from your rib cage to your pubic bone. When it contracts, it brings your pelvis toward your chest and/or your chest toward your pelvis, depending on your position at the time.

In order to demonstrate this to yourself, lie on the floor on your back with your knees bent and your feet lifted in the air. Place your fingers of both hands just below your belly button and your thumbs just below your breastbone. Now press the small of your back against the floor and gently roll your pelvis up toward your chest. You will feel your rectus abdominis contract.

Other muscles of the abdominal wall are the "internal" and "external obliques," which are on each side of the rectus abdominis. The external oblique goes diagonally from the front inside top of your hip to the outside of your lower ribs. This may sound confusing, but if you take the left (or the right) hand and place it on the same side between your hip and your ribs, with your fingers angled slightly down toward and near your belly button, you will get the idea of where the external oblique muscle is and in which direction it runs. When this muscle contracts it causes rotation of the trunk, bringing the rib cage *in* toward the rectus abdominis. With your right hand on the muscle on your right side, rotate your torso to the left, and you will feel how the external oblique muscle contracts. (If you rotate to the right, the muscle on the left side will be working.)

The internal oblique lies underneath the external oblique (that is, farther inside you). It runs diagonally, in the opposite direction from the external obliques. It goes from the inside front of the ribs, back and down to the outside of the hip. You can locate this muscle if you place your right hand on your left side. Put your index finger on the crest of your hip and angle your hand up so the wrist is above your belly button and the thumb runs along the bottom of the ribs. Remember the external oblique is on top of the internal oblique, so you may not be able to feel it contract—but here is how it works. With your right hand placed on the internal oblique on your left side, twist to the left, and you should be able to feel the muscle contract to cause the movement.

The last muscle of the abdominal wall is the "transverse abdominis." It is a broad sheet of muscle underneath the other three abdominal muscles, and it covers virtually your entire abdominal area. This muscle pulls the other abdominal muscles in toward the spine and helps stabilize the trunk, but unlike the other abdominal muscles, its contraction does not result in a movement that rotates or flexes the spine. Because it is underneath the other abdominal muscles, it is the hardest one to feel with your hand, but if you press softly on your abdomen and cough, you may be able to feel it working. It also contracts when you exhale or laugh hard.

The Movements of the Midsection and Ab Exercises

There are four movements the trunk or midsection can make. "Flexion," which means bending forward or rounding your lower back, is caused by the rectus abdominis, and secondarily by the outer obliques. "Lateral flexion" is leaning your shoulder to the side, toward your hip, from the waist, and is made possible by the inner and outer obliques. "Rotation"

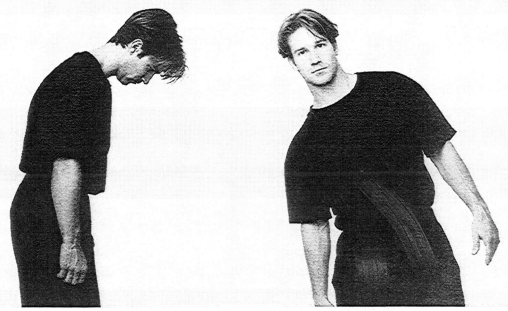

Flexion   Lateral flexion

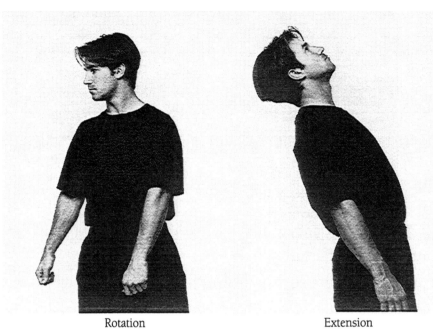

Rotation   Extension

is twisting the midsection to either side, as if you were to look behind you by turning from the waist; it also involves the inner and outer obliques. "Extension" is bending backward or arching your back. It stretches the abdominal wall but it is not caused by your ab muscles, instead it is made possible by the muscles of the low back.

The Body-Mind Connection

All exercises for your abs involve only those four muscles and those three simple movements. As you do an exercise, it helps if you actually visualize which muscles and movements are involved, and exactly how the muscles are working to cause the movements.

When you do ab exercises, don't think about lunch or what work you need to do. Instead, focus your mind on the muscles working in any particular exercise and visualize them contracting to make the movement. The brain and the muscles work together, so if you think about which muscle you're working, you'll be able to isolate and strengthen it more effectively by doing the movement completely and correctly. You'll be less likely to recruit other, superfluous muscles—such as those in your legs or your neck when you do a crunch—which will do absolutely zero for your abs.

Pregnancy and Abs

When you become pregnant, your baby grows inside your uterus, located behind the lower part of the abdominal wall. Remember that muscles are adaptable so they can stretch? Well, pregnancy is when your abs *really* stretch. They will still feel tight because the uterus is expanding behind and pushing against them. Unfortunately, this tightness is deceptive in that it does not necessarily mean your ab muscles are well conditioned.

You can tone the muscles of the abdominal area during pregnancy, as we show you in chapter three. They just have to work around the fetus instead of across the normal surface.

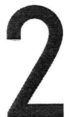

2 PREGNANCY AND EXERCISE

It wasn't so long ago that when a woman became pregnant she was advised to minimize her physical activity. Such advice was based on the intuition she should play it safe or, perhaps, on Victorian notions of pregnancy as a "delicate condition," but it wasn't backed up by much medical research. In fact, not until the past 10 years or so has any reliable scientific work been done on the effects of exercise on pregnant women and their fetuses.

In 1994 the American College of Obstetricians and Gynecologists (ACOG) issued *Recommendations for Exercise in Pregnancy and Postpartum,* which state: "During pregnancy, women can continue to exercise and derive health benefits even from mild-to-moderate exercise." Recent studies continue to show that exercise during pregnancy helps alleviate some of the more common prenatal complaints you might have—including varicose veins, leg cramps and swelling, and constipation—and also contributes to fewer complications during labor. Exercise will probably help you sleep better and improve your mood generally. It will help you avoid putting on more weight than you need. There is even evidence to suggest if you perform regular aerobic exercise during pregnancy, you may give birth to a bigger, healthier baby.

Exercise during pregnancy has another benefit I have seen time and time again among my clients. Those women who are fit before pregnancy, and who continue to stay fit during pregnancy, bounce back into top shape very quickly after childbirth. By contrast, those women who come to me only after childbirth have to work harder and longer to get back into shape.

Developing strong abdominal muscles before you get pregnant and maintaining them during pregnancy are two of the biggest gifts you can give yourself. Strong abs will support your growing fetus better, and they will help relieve the low-back pain that you may experience from supporting all that extra weight in your midsection. The purpose of any fitness program during pregnancy is to create such health benefits. Body-shaping, weight loss, and setting records for endurance or strength are *not* appropriate goals during this period— and the idea of maintaining a flat stomach with a fetus growing inside you is clearly absurd. There's a lot of pressure on women in our society to look like rail-thin fashion models. If you bought this book, you are clearly the kind of person who is concerned about her appearance. But during pregnancy, as your waistline expands, you've really got to resist any negative feelings about your appearance. Just think of Demi Moore, who celebrated the beautiful body of a woman with child by posing for the cover of *Vanity Fair* when she was 8 months pregnant. And the idea that you'll never be as trim and taut as you were is ridiculous. I work with many women athletes and fitness professionals, and I'm always amazed at how fast they snap back into top condition—often within months. These women are at the top end of the fitness spectrum—but the same principles of exercise and diet will work for you, too.

When Exercise Is Not Recommended

Before undertaking or continuing any exercise program during pregnancy, you must discuss it with your doctor or healthcare provider and get her approval. There are still certain complications that may cause your doctor to advise against exercise. In those cases you must follow her advice. After a safe childbirth, you *will* be able to get back into shape.

There are certain cases in which exercise during pregnancy is definitely not recommended. According to ACOG these are

> pregnancy-induced hypertension
>
> preterm rupture of membranes
>
> preterm labor during the prior or current pregnancy or both
>
> incompetent cervix/cerclage
>
> persistent second- or third-trimester bleeding
>
> intrauterine growth retardation
>
> multiple gestation (twins, triplets, et al.)

ACOG also advises special care and consultation with your doctor or healthcare giver if you have the following conditions: chronic hypertension or overactive thyroid; or cardiac, vascular, or pulmonary disease.

Warning Signs to Stop Exercising

If any of the following signs occur during exercise, you should stop immediately and get in touch with your doctor or healthcare provider:

Pain in the hips, legs, pubic area, abdomen, or chest

Any bleeding or discharge from the vagina

Headache, lightheadedness, faintness, or dizziness

More shortness of breath than usual*

Sudden swelling in the hands, feet, or face

Fever or overheating

Nausea or vomiting

Uterine contractions

Heart palpitations

Which Sports and Fitness Activities Are Considered Safe During Pregnancy?

Many of the fitness activities you enjoy are considered safe during pregnancy—with some modifications. Here is a list with guidelines:

Running	reduce intensity; avoid overheating and dehydration
Cycling	avoid conditions where spills are likely, such as wet pavement, unpaved roads, congested areas, heavy traffic, etc.
Swimming	don't dive or jump into the water; no frog kicks
Aerobics	low impact only
Cross-country skiing	Avoid icy conditions, large hills, or high altitudes (above 10,000 feet)
Weight training	Be careful of low-back strain; see warning below about exercising on back after first trimester
Racquet sports	reduce intensity; switch to doubles in tennis; stop after second trimester

*It is common for pregnant women to feel short of breath in pregnancy due to high progesterone levels and musculoskeletal changes. The enlarged uterus pushes the diaphragm up so that it cannot be used as effectively for respiration.

Which Sports and Fitness Activities Are Considered Unsafe?

All contact sports (football, rugby, etc.), downhill skiing, water-skiing, inline skating, ice skating, scuba diving, diving, surfing, skydiving, hang gliding, gymnastics, horseback riding, mountain- and rock-climbing, strenuous hiking at high altitudes, and mountain biking on rough terrain are not advised. Use common sense here—anything that puts you at risk of trauma or falling should be avoided. In general, I don't recommend competitive sports such as basketball, soccer, and field hockey because you are more apt to get caught up in the excitement of the moment and forget about being cautious.

Watch Your Balance

Your body undergoes enormous changes during pregnancy. As your uterus grows to *1,000 times* its normal size, you gain on an average of 18 to 26 pounds (or more), and your breasts enlarge, your center of gravity shifts. This will become especially evident in the second and third trimesters, when you put on most of the weight. As a result, you must be careful not to lose your balance. Never do any activities that will place

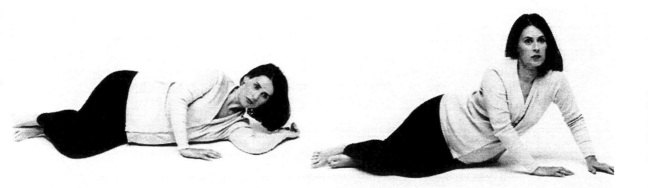

The correct way to get up from lying on your side.

you at risk of losing your balance. Always get up slowly from a lying or sitting position, and make sure there is something around to hold on to in case you feel dizzy.

Be Careful of Sprains and Injuries—Your Hormones Are Working Overtime

As your body prepares for childbirth, it experiences a dramatic rise in the level of certain hormones—in particular, estrogen, progesterone, and relaxin. These make your joints and ligaments softer, more flexible—and progressively more susceptible to injury and strain. Remember this when you are stretching—resist the temptation to go too far and over-stretch. In addition avoid making any sudden, jerky movements.

The Danger of Overheating

Overheating is dangerous both for you and your fetus, particularly during the first trimester. Your core temperature should not exceed 100.4 degrees F (38 degrees C). You should not exercise in very hot or humid weather unless you're inside with air-conditioning. Drink plenty of liquids and wear cool, loose-fitting clothing. Don't exercise if you have a fever, and don't use saunas or hot tubs. Don't continue exercising until you feel exhausted. If you feel fatigued or exhausted, stop immediately.

Forget about high-intensity, rigorous exercise during pregnancy. If you are a fitness devotee or an elite athlete, take down the intensity of your workouts several notches. Stop trying to make performance gains until you've regained your strength and stamina after childbirth.

Obviously you are not going to exercise with a thermometer in your mouth—but if you do start to feel feverish, stop and take your temperature. During pregnancy, your target heart rate range is 60 percent to 75 percent. On page 55 I give you the standard method for determining your heart rate. It may seem a little complicated and fussy at first, but once you do it a couple of times, you'll see that it's no big deal.

Competitive athletes and fitness trainers do it all the time.

Probably the easiest method for determining the proper level of exertion is the Rate of Perceived Exertion, or RPE scale, which you will find on page 55. It is a method for codifying your gut feeling about how hard you are working out. During pregnancy you should not be exerting yourself over 13—registering no more than "somewhat hard."

A good method to use in conjunction with the RPE scale is the "talk test." It's simple: at all times during exercise, you should easily be able to carry on a conversation, without gasping or pausing for breath.

Exercising on Your Back After the First Trimester

ACOG does not recommend exercising on your back after the first trimester. The reason is "supine hypotensive syndrome," which can occur when the weight of your enlarged uterus puts too much pressure on a major blood vein (the inferior vena cava). This is a problem especially with vigorous exercise performed while you are on your back. The symptoms are dizziness, nausea, and difficulty in breathing—and you can even pass out.

From experience with my clients, I find that this problem has been a bit overexaggerated. Some women are so freaked out about the prospect of it that when they wake up at night on their backs, they worry that they might have harmed their baby.

Hypotensive supine syndrome is actually not a problem for many women. Of all the pregnant clients I've had over the years and all the pregnant women I've talked to, I've met only a few who have experienced it! (Actually my mom tells me she did.) This is not to say that it is not a problem—just that it is not universal.

The symptoms are easy to recognize because they come on gradually. So if you find you have a problem, you'll have plenty of time to do something about it. If you are on your back and any of the above symptoms appear, roll gently onto your left side and breathe normally until you feel better. There is little danger that you will harm your fetus.

Many ab exercises, such as crunches, are performed on your back.

Unless you find you are experiencing supine hypotensive syndrome or are a particularly nervous sort, there's no need to give up completely in your second and third trimesters. But you should take a few precautions: when lying on your back, reduce the intensity of all exercises, and don't spend more than 5 minutes exercising on your back at any one time. Of course if you do find you start feeling the symptoms, abandon any exercising on your back. In the next chapter I give ab exercises performed in other positions for those who have the problem, or those who are simply not comfortable risking the possibility of it.

If I Wasn't Exercising Before I Was Pregnant, Can I Start Now that I Am?

If you don't have any of the conditions that contraindicate exercise and if your doctor or medical caregiver approves, there is no reason you can't start a gentle exercise program during pregnancy. To be on the safe side, wait until the second trimester, when the danger of overheating is a bit less serious. I would particularly recommend walking and swimming in a pool for your aerobic exercise.

Some Other Tips for Exercise During Pregnancy

Exercise regularly. In order to reap the benefits of exercise, you must do it regularly—preferably at least 3 times a week. Pregnancy and the period after childbirth are periods when you have many demands on your time and other things on your mind. You will find that you become fatigued more easily and may be tempted to skip your workout. But sporadic exercise will do you little good and may even place you at higher risk for injury. So make a realistic plan, and stick to it.

Eat a piece of fruit an hour before you exercise. Morning sickness occurs in more than half of all pregnancies, typically during the first

3 months. The symptoms are worse on an empty stomach. Many women find that if they eat an apple, orange, or banana an hour before they work out, they have more energy and are less prone to become so nauseated that they abandon all thought of exercise. Another helpful hint is to get outside in the fresh air—a traditional remedy for alleviating nausea.

Get new athletic shoes. Talk to the clerk at your local athletic store and get the right shoes for your sport: cross-training shoes for aerobics, running shoes for jogging, etc. The appropriate footwear can be invaluable in helping you keep your balance and avoid injuries.

Get a sports bra. During pregnancy your breasts will enlarge, and, especially in the first months, become tender and sensitive. Be sure to get a comfortable sports bra that offers adequate support. Because your breasts will probably continue to get bigger throughout your pregnancy, you may have to buy new bras when the old ones get too tight. Even though this can be a rather expensive proposition, you should do this rather than wear one that causes discomfort—your bra should not be so tight that it leaves any marks on your skin.

Your breast size will most likely plateau around the eighth month. When you buy a bra then, make sure there is a little extra room because your breasts will probably enlarge somewhat additionally when your milk comes in. It is especially important when you are breastfeeding that your bra not be too tight because that can cause clogged milk ducts. You may want to look into buying a bra specifically designed for breastfeeding.

Drink plenty of water. It's always a good idea to drink 6 to 8 glasses of water daily, but especially crucial in helping to avoid prenatal overheating.

Don't get too far away from a bathroom. As your uterus enlarges it puts pressure on your bladder. Many women find that exercise, especially, causes a need for frequent urination. Go to the bathroom before you start exercising and make repeat visits as often as you need to. *Do not* restrict your intake of fluids—this will only cause dehydration and aggravate any feelings of nausea you may have.

Listen to Your Body and Use Common Sense

Much of the advice for working out during pregnancy is pretty much common sense—so make sure you bring that with you to your workouts. If any activity feels unsafe or risky, don't do it. If your body doesn't feel right, stop what you are doing and check with your doctor. And always bear in mind these cardinal rules:

- Get permission from your doctor or medical caregiver

- Watch your balance

- Don't overheat or overexert

- Be mindful of any unusual symptoms and stop if you experience any

- Don't overstretch or make jerky movements that put you at risk for muscle strains

- Be careful about exercising on your back after the first trimester

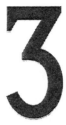

3 MIDSECTION STRETCHES AND EXERCISES DURING PREGNANCY

When you are pregnant you need to change your mindset about ab exercises rather dramatically. You're not trying to maintain a flat midsection here. You're doing ab exercises solely for the health benefits—to keep your ab muscles toned, to help you maintain better posture, to help alleviate the stress of the weight of the fetus and enlarged uterus on your low back, and to aid in an easier delivery and recovery afterward.

As I said in the last chapter, if you are a regular exerciser and your doctor gives permission, you can continue your usual ab routine, at least during the first trimester—that is, unless you have been performing the U.S. Marine Corps system or something similarly fanatical. In that case you'll need to tone down the intensity. As you get bigger (which happens at different times for different women), you'll naturally want to take it easier, as well as to omit those exercises that are becoming awkward—such as reverse crunches (see page 77) and oblique crunches (see page 75). Remember to avoid the danger of overheating, especially during the first trimester.

Can I Begin an Ab Routine During Pregnancy If I Never Did One Before?

If you weren't exercising before you became pregnant, you may begin a gentle program, with the permission of your doctor or medical caregiver. For the first trimester, at least, I recommend going to Month 1 Easy of the abdominal exercises in chapter seven (see pages 67–71). There you will learn how to do abdominal contractions, pelvic tilts, simple crunches, and side bends. For the second and third trimesters go to the midsection stretches on pages 24–29 and pick two or three ab exercises from those on pages 29–34. Wait until after you recover from childbirth before going on to the more strenuous ab exercises.

Proper Technique for Ab Exercises

You always need to do exercises with proper technique in order to get the full benefits and to avoid injury. Perform stretches and abdominal exercises on a mat, thick carpet, or other soft flooring (a good idea even when you're not pregnant). Don't hold your breath during exercise: The reduced amount of oxygen to your brain could cause light-headedness or fainting. Always breathe normally. If you are a first-time ab exerciser, I want to give you detailed instructions about proper technique in the descriptions in chapter seven of the Month 1 Easy ab exercises I recommend above.

If you are a regular exerciser continuing with your own routine, I'd like you also to review proper technique for ab exercises here. It is all too easy to get a bit sloppy and careless when you've been doing something for a while and it becomes rote.

1. Always use a slow, controlled movement throughout the entire range of motion in an exercise. Never jerk up, make sudden movements, or let momentum or gravity carry you through.

2. When you exercise your abs, focus the entire movement on your abs. You should not feel strain in other muscles, such as those in your low back or neck. If you do, go back and check your form.

3. Never hold your breath. Breathe properly. Exhale slowly as you perform the harder part of the movement—on the way up in a crunch, for instance. This will cause your abs to contract even more than they would normally. Inhale slowly as you go back to the starting position.

4. Keep the tension on the muscle you are working throughout an entire exercise. Do this by not pausing at the starting position between each repetition. Remember, if you relax the muscle, you are not making it work.

The All-Important Pelvic Floor Muscles

The pelvic floor (PF) muscles form a figure 8 around the anus, the vagina, and the urethra. The PF muscles are important for several reasons, even though they aren't abdominal muscles. Like a sack or a sling, the PF muscles support the weight of everything in the pelvic area—in particular, the uterus, the bladder, and the bowel. They control bowel and bladder activity. They aid in sexual pleasure. And they are very important during childbirth, when they must relax and stretch in order to let the baby out.

During pregnancy the increased weight of the fetus and the uterus can cause your pelvic floor muscles to stretch and sag. So, you must strengthen your pelvic floor muscles through special exercises called Kegels. They are simple to do, but their importance can't be overestimated. It is best if you begin doing Kegels while you are pregnant—or even before—because after childbirth the muscles are so stretched that you may find it difficult to locate them and to learn the feel of the exercises.

To locate your pelvic floor muscles, pretend you are stopping a stream of urine. You'll feel the muscles in the whole area—the sphincter, the vagina, and the urethra—contract. Notice that you can contract them slightly or you can make them very tight.

To perform a Kegel exercise contract your pelvic floor muscles as tightly as is comfortably possible and hold for 3 to 5 seconds. Rest for 2 to 3 seconds, then make the contraction again. Repeat this 5 times. Throughout an entire day do 10 sets of 5 repetitions each. Do a set when you're driving, or when you're talking on the phone, or when a commercial comes on the television. You can do Kegels any time and in any position—when you're talking to your mother-in-law, say—and no one will be the wiser for it. Do a set at the beginning of your exercise session and another at the end.

You'll be surprised how fast these muscles get stronger through exercise. After just a few days you'll be able to feel the difference. You'll appreciate the change next time you have to urinate, because you'll have a far easier time making it to the bathroom comfortably. And strong pelvic floor muscles will increase your pleasure during sex—and probably your husband's as well. Try practicing a few Kegels while your husband or lover is inside you.

As your pelvic floor muscles get stronger, you can refine your Kegel technique. Try holding each one for 10 to 20 seconds. Or try what is often called "elevator" Kegels. Pretend you are riding in an elevator and as you ascend each floor, make your pelvic floor muscles a little tighter. When they're as tight as you can make them (and you're on the imaginary top floor), go back down floor by floor, releasing a little bit each time.

Incidentally, men can do Kegels too. They may be a little skeptical at first, but next time one of your male friends has had a couple of beers and there's a long line at the bathroom, he'll thank you if he took your advice to do the exercises. A man can also increase his (and your) sexual pleasure by doing Kegels. Supposedly they are the heart of the ancient

Arabic discipline of *Imsak*, in which men learn to pinch off and delay their orgasm for hours so they can prolong their lovemaking and drive lovers wild. Wow! That should be enough incentive for you and your husband or lover to start doing Kegels tonight!

Diastasis Recti

Some pregnant women experience a painless condition called "diastasis recti," which usually starts in the second trimester, where the two sides of the rectus abdominis (you'll remember from chapter two that this is the long band of muscle that runs from the ribs to the pelvis) separate down the middle. This is your body's way of preventing the muscle from stretching too far because of your enlarging uterus. The condition is generally harmless and you can easily correct it through a special exercise after childbirth—we'll show you how in chapter five (see page 46). However, because it weakens abdominal muscles, it calls for modifications to your abdominal routine. Many regular ab exercises such as crunches pull on the sides of the rectus, so performing them will cause the separation to get bigger. *During pregnancy (and in the first weeks after childbirth) you need to check for a separation before each workout with the test described below.*

Self-Test for Diastasis Recti

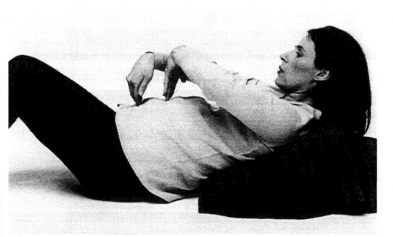

Lie on your back on the floor with your knees bent and your feet flat on the floor. Lift your head and bring your chin to your chest. Find the vertical ridge of muscle that runs down the center of your abdomen. With your fingertips pointing down, toward the floor, and your palms toward your face, press firmly just above and just below your navel into the soft, vertical gap in the middle. If the separation is greater than one inch (two-fingers width) you should do only the following special ab exercise. It will prevent the muscle from separating further, while keeping your abs toned.

Special Exercise for Diastasis Recti

Lie on your back with your legs bent and your feet flat on the floor. (If you are having a problem with supine hypotensive syndrome—see page 14—use a pillow or two to elevate your head and shoulders above the midsection.) Place your right hand on the left side of your rectus abdominis and your left hand on the right side. Your hands will be crossed, one over the other, and your fingertips will be on each side of your bellybutton, pointing out toward your sides. Now, exhale slowly, pull the two sides of your rectus together, lift your head off the floor, and move your chin toward your chest. Keep your shoulders on the floor, and don't jerk up. The higher you can lift your head, the more your abs

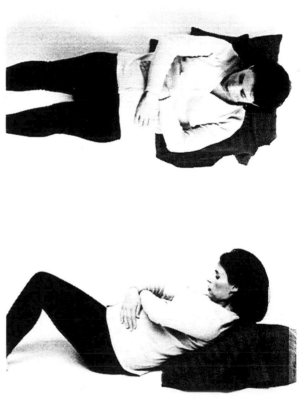

will engage. Pause for a count of 2, holding the two sides of your rectus firmly together with your fingertips the whole time, then return slowly to the floor and repeat. Do 1 set of 5 reps, 2 or 3 times a day— perhaps in bed, 1 set before you get up in the morning and another before you go to sleep at night.

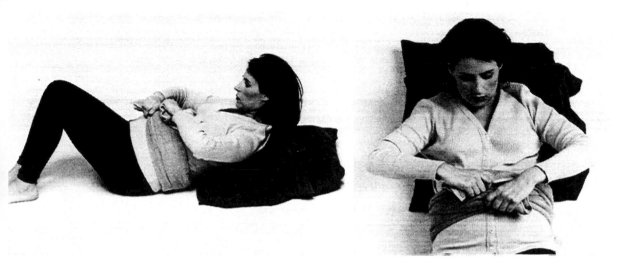

There is an alternate method of holding the two sides of your rectus abdominis together that you may prefer. Get a towel and wrap it around your waist, below your ribs and above your hips. Get in the position described above. Hold the right side of the towel with your left hand and the left side of the towel with your right, so the two ends cross. Now pull each side with light tension as you raise your head slowly. Remember to maintain the pressure on both sides of the towel throughout the exercise.

You'll notice that the above exercise is performed while lying on your back, a position not recommended by ACOG after the first trimester. Because the exercise takes a minute or so and it's very gentle, you shouldn't have a problem. If you do, however, you can place 2 or 3 pillows under your shoulders to elevate them above your midsection for the exercise. Then proceed as above: bring your chin to your chest and contract your abs as you pull them together with your hands or a towel.

Stretching Your Abs and Lower Back During the Pregnant Months

It's always a good idea to stretch, but especially so during pregnancy because the weight gain and changes in your body place so much stress on your lower back. Here are some good stretches for your abdomen and lower back during pregnancy. They will help to relieve any lower-back pain you experience, and also enable you to maintain a fuller range of motion and better posture.

Perform these stretches before and after you exercise, and perhaps also in the morning soon after you get up. You can do them anytime you are feeling tight and tired—because they will help refresh you.

I. Lower Back Stretch/Strengthen

You may be one of the many women who experience a weakened lower back during pregnancy. Here is a good exercise to stretch and strengthen it so it will be in balance with your abdominal muscles. Sit in a chair with your legs bent at 90 degrees and your feet flat on the floor. Sit up straight—shoulders relaxed, down, and back—then round forward, bringing your head toward your

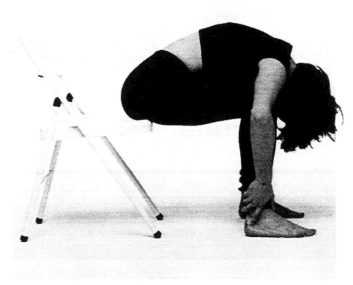

knees, as far as is comfortable, until you feel a comfortable stretch in your lower back. Try to pull yourself down a little farther by taking hold of your ankles, and exhale as you do so. Suck your abs in at the bottom of the movement. Then, breathing normally, slowly return to the upright position. At the top, arch your back slightly and pull your shoulder blades back down and together. Hold this position for a second then repeat the exercise. Try to do 2 sets of 10 slow repetitions.

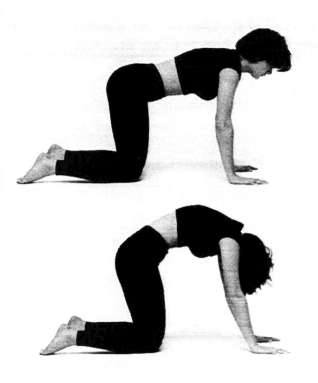

2. The Cat Stretch

Get down on the floor on your hands and knees. Exhale and round your lower back, pushing the small of your back—not your shoulder blades—up toward the ceiling. Relax your neck and shoulders as your head goes down. Hold the position for 5 seconds, then inhale and slowly go back to the starting position—so that your back is slightly arched, as in the photo.

3. Hip Swings

In the same starting position as the Cat Stretch—on your hands and knees with a slight arch in your lower back—and without moving your legs, slowly twist your right hip toward your right shoulder, as far as is comfortable, and hold for 2 seconds. Then go back to center and repeat with your left hip toward your left shoulder. Make certain you move only your hips in this exercise and not your shoulders. This will stretch the muscles between your hips and your ribs. It also moves your spine from side to side, which should feel good.

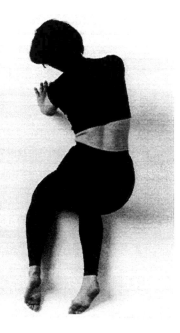

4. "The Pose of the Child" or "The Folded Leaf"

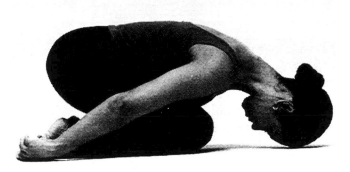

This stretch is from yoga. Kneel on the floor with your toes pointed back behind you. Lower your butt to your ankles and round your back forward so your chest is on your thighs. Reach your hands back toward the bottoms of your feet. Duck your chin down toward your your chest as much as possible. Hold this position for 20 to 30 seconds, rest, then repeat. This is a great stretch for your lower back and the tailbone area. Many women who have just given birth particularly like this stretch. During pregnancy, when your belly gets big, don't sit on your ankles; instead, position your knees and ankles out wider than your hips.

5. Hip and Butt Stretch

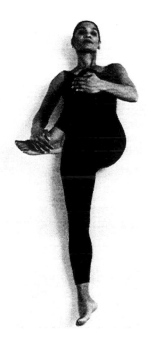

Lie on the floor on your back, legs out straight. Raise your right leg so the knee bends and comes across your body toward the left shoulder. Grab the right knee with your right hand and the ankle with the left hand. Gently pull both the knee and the ankle across the body, stretching the back and outside of your hip area. Hold a comfortable stretch for 20 seconds, then do the other side. You can do this stretch until your belly gets too big to pull your leg over. If you have a problem with supine hypotensive syndrome, omit this stretch or use pillows to elevate your shoulders above your midsection.

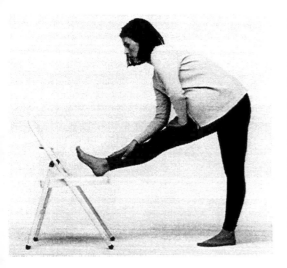

6. Standing hamstring stretch

Put a sturdy table or chair that is knee-height tall next to a wall. Stand next to the wall and in front of the chair. Put your right heel up on the chair, with your knee straight and locked out. Holding on to the wall with the hand nearest it for balance, bend forward from your hips until you feel a mild tension in the back of your right leg. Breathe normally, keep your back straight and head up. Hold for at least 20 seconds, then repeat with your left leg up on the chair.

7. Standing Torso Twists

Stand with your feet shoulder-width apart and your knees unlocked. Turn easily from side to side, rotating from your waist and not your hips, which should stay square to whatever you're facing. Keep your neck still so your head and shoulders move together. Perform two 30-second sets.

8. Hip Circles

Stand with your feet shoulder-width apart, knees slightly bent, and your hands just above your hips. For 30 seconds rotate your hips easily in small circles, then gradually increase the size of the circles but not beyond your comfort range. Then repeat in the other direction.

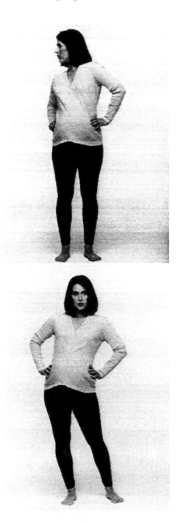

9. Supported Squats

With both hands grab onto something that is sturdy and immovable, like the back of a couch, which is about 2–3 feet off the floor. Or have a partner hold you firmly by both hands with your arms fully extended. With your feet a little wider than your shoulders, and your toes turned out, squat down as far as is comfortable. Sit back into the stretch for 30 seconds.

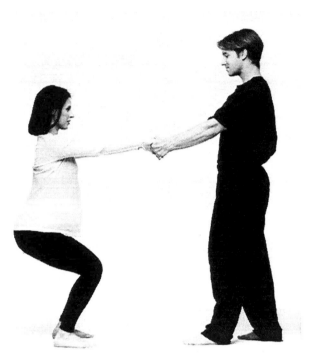

Second- and Third-Trimester Ab and Lower Back Exercises

As I said in chapter two, ACOG and some prenatal fitness professionals advise against exercising on your back after the first trimester because of supine hypotensive syndrome. Again, as a fitness professional who has worked with many pregnant women, I want to assure you that many women do not experience the problem. If you are one of the women not affected by it, you can continue with back-lying ab exercises, such as those found in the System, while taking the precautions of *not exercising too vigorously and not spending more than 5 minutes exercising on your back at any one time.* If you do find yourself experiencing any of the symptoms—nausea, dizziness, difficulty breathing—gently roll onto your left side (which will shift the weight of the uterus off the vena cava) and lie there until the symptoms subside. Also, as with the ab exercise for diastasis recti, you can place two or three pillows under your shoulders to elevate them.

For women who do experience the problem, or for those who are simply nervous about it, there are ab-toning exercises that are not performed on your back. Even if you don't experience supine hypotensive syndrome, you may find these exercises more comfortable than the traditional ones during the final weeks of pregnancy.

1. Standing Pelvic Tilt

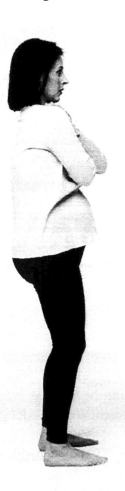

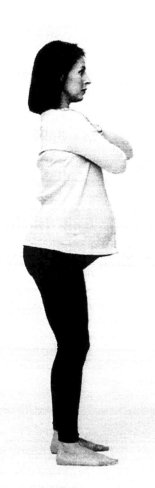

Stand with your back against a wall, so your shoulder blades and buttocks touch the wall. Or simply stand straight without any support. Your knees should be slightly bent, your feet shoulder-width apart, and about 12 inches away from the wall, if you are using one. Take a deep breath and as you exhale, slowly rotate your pelvis up so the small of your back presses back or against the wall; simultaneously tighten your abdominal muscles. Hold for a count of 3; relax and repeat 10 times.

2. Seated Abdominal Contractions

Sit on the floor with your legs crossed and, if you like, with your entire back against a wall for support. Relax your arms at your sides. Take a deep breath and as you exhale pull your bellybutton in so your abdominals contract and the small of your back flattens, against the wall if you are using one. Hold that position for five seconds then relax and take another deep breath. Do this 10 times, then rest for 30 seconds and do another set of 10.

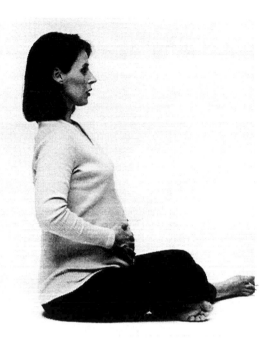

3. Ab Contractions on All Fours

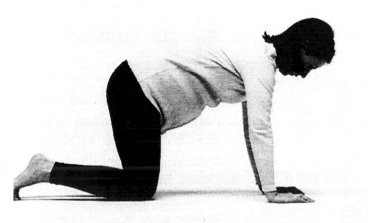

This is the same movement as the Cat Stretch on page 26, but here you focus on your abs tightening instead of your back stretching. Get down on your hands and knees, with your hands under your shoulders and your knees under your hips. Keep your back flat, don't let it sag. Take a deep breath. Then, as you exhale slowly, press the small of your back (*not* your shoulder blades) toward the ceiling as you contract your abdominals. Hold for a count of 3 and then relax to the starting position. Repeat 10 times.

4. Opposite Arm and Leg Raise on All Fours

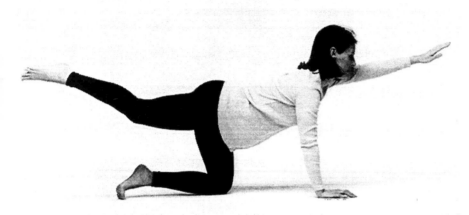

This exercise is for strengthening your butt and your low back—so that's where you should feel it. Get down on your hands and knees, hands under your shoulders, knees under your hips. As in the previous exercise, make sure to keep your back flat—don't arch it too much. Take a deep breath and, as you slowly exhale, tighten your abdominals. Raise your right arm, reaching it out straight in front of you; at the same time, extend your left leg straight out behind. Hold for 1 second, then slowly return to the starting position. Do 10 repetitions, then do 10 more with the left arm and right leg.

5. Hip and Shoulder Crunch

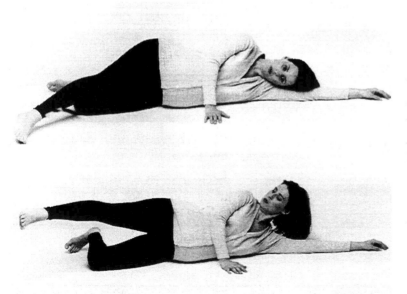

Lie on your side with your bottom leg bent slightly and your bottom arm extended out above your head, palm on the floor. Rest your head on the bottom arm and put the palm of your other arm on the floor in front of you for support. Now, inhale and extend your top leg out straight, a few inches off the floor. As you exhale, crunch the top of your hip toward your top shoulder and, at the same time, bring the shoulder toward the hip. Hold for 1 or 2 seconds and then relax in the starting position. This is a slight movement, but you should be able to feel the muscles on the side of your abs working. Do 10 repetitions and then repeat, lying on your other side.

Ab Exercises in a Pool

Many women find that exercising in a pool is easier than on dry land when they are pregnant. The buoyancy of water makes you lighter and more comfortable. For these exercises stand in chest-deep water and use the side of the pool for support.

I. Standing Pelvic Tilts

Perform as on page 30 with your back against the side of the pool. Do at least 10 reps and more if you like.

2. Reverse Crunch, Alternating Legs

Float on your stomach while grasping the pool edge with one hand and putting the other against the pool wall for support. As you take a deep breath in (don't swallow any pool water!), exhale, contract your abs, and slowly pull one leg toward your chest. Then slowly straighten your leg and return to the starting position. Repeat with the other leg. Do 3 sets of 10, taking at least a minute for each set.

3. Reverse Crunch, Both Legs

Perform as above, but pull both legs to your chest at the same time. Do 3 sets of 10.

4. Side Bends

Stand in chest-deep water, with your back against the pool wall for balance. Let your arms hang at your sides. Sliding your right hand down your right thigh, bring your right shoulder toward your right hip. Bend as far as is comfortable and don't bend forward or backward from the waist. Return slowly to the starting position. Then perform the exercise to the left. Do 3 sets of 10 to both sides.

Summing Up the Basics of a Pregnancy Ab Routine

- Get the approval of your doctor or medical caregiver to start or continue with exercise.

- Be careful not to overheat, especially during the first trimester. Always make sure you pass the "talk test" (see page 14) while exercising.

- Do ab exercises every other day. Your muscles need 48 hours to recover from each exercise session. It's a good idea to alternate ab exercise days with aerobic exercise days.

- Remind yourself always that your goal is toning your ab muscles for the health benefits—*not* body shaping or maintaining a flat midsection.

- Stretch your abs and lower back gently before and after each ab session.

- Check for diastasis recti before each workout. If the gap is greater than one inch, you must do only the special exercise for diastasis on page 23. The gap usually develops after the first trimester, but some women have a gap that never completely closed from a previous pregnancy.

- For your first trimester, continue with your regular ab routine, decreasing the intensity, or to go to Month 1 Easy of the System. Whatever your ab routine, it should not take longer than 10 minutes to complete, not including stretches.

- If you have a problem with supine hypotensive syndrome or are uncomfortable on your back, switch to ab exercises that don't require lying on your back, given above.

- As your pregnancy gets further along and your belly gets bigger, tone down your ab routine even further. Women differ so in their fitness levels and the progressions of their pregnancies that it's difficult to tell you exactly when to do this—but as athletes like to say, listen to your body. If it doesn't feel good, stop doing it. For the final months, choose 2 or 3 of the exercises above that don't require lying on your back and do 1 to 3 sets of 10 repetitions for each exercise.

4 A WORD ON PREGNANCY, DIET, AND WEIGHT GAIN

Even if you are considerably overweight, your doctor or medical caregiver will tell you not to diet while you are pregnant. The reason is that you risk not getting essential nutrients that your fetus needs. For instance, a deficiency of folic acid (found in dark-green leafy vegetables, oranges, lentils, pinto and lima beans, peanuts, cashews) has been linked to neural-tube defects, such as spina bifida; calcium (in milk, cheese, dark-green leafy vegetables, dried beans and peas) is crucial for fetal-bone development; vitamin C (citrus fruit, green peppers, strawberries) is necessary for forming skin and tendons; iron (red meat, fish, poultry, whole grains, dark-green leafy vegetables) for making red blood cells and so forth.

These days doctors usually advise women to gain between 24 and 35 pounds during pregnancy (some underweight women may be told to put on more, overweight women less). This was not always the case. My mom was told in the early seventies when she was pregnant with me that if she put on more than 15 pounds her obstetrician wouldn't even see her. The thinking then was that a bigger fetus increased a women's chances of complications during childbirth—including cesarean births, which are more often necessary for bigger babies. Since that time, important studies found that low birth weight (which is related to the mother's weight—big women have big babies and vice versa) was a factor in infant mortality.

However, weight gain in pregnancy seems to be one of those issues for which the pendulum swings back and forth. In 1998 a study published in the *New England Journal of Medicine*, led by Dr. Sven Cnattingius of the Karolinska Institute in Stockholm, looked at more than 167,000 Swedish women and found that lean women had far fewer stillbirths and infant deaths in the first week after birth than did normal and overweight women. The babies of obese women were at greatest risk—these women were four times as likely to have a stillbirth with their first child than lean women were. The study concluded that ". . . pregnancies among lean women should be regarded as characterized by a low rather than a high risk of adverse outcome. . . . Advising lean women to gain weight before becoming pregnant may not be justified."

Clearly there is more scientific work to be done in this area, but for now the best course for pregnant women seems to be to gain the weight your doctor or medical caregiver recommends but no more. Of course, prenatal weight gain is highly individual. Many women tell me that they have an instinctive feeling about how much they should eat, and how much weight they need to gain during pregnancy—and that this can differ even for the same woman in different pregnancies. The important thing is that you put on the weight the right way, by eating nutritious foods that supply you with the protein, vitamin C, folic acid, iron, calcium, and other essential nutritional building blocks that you and your fetus need.

You should *not* use pregnancy as *carte blanche* to gorge on food you would never dream of eating otherwise: ice-cream sundaes, macaroni and cheese, fudge by the pan. The problem is that junk food contains empty calories, i.e., few of the nutrients you and your fetus need. The foods you should be eating—fresh fruits and vegetables, whole grains, lean red meat, poultry, and fish—are not loaded with fat, refined sugar, and artificial ingredients. It doesn't take a genius to figure out that foods not good for you normally aren't any better for you during pregnancy.

Remember that fat does not magically disappear after childbirth. If you put on a lot more weight than your doctor recommends, you will be stuck with it after the baby comes. As you monitor your weight during pregnancy, remember that most of the gain comes later rather than sooner: during the first trimester you will probably gain only 2 to 4 pounds. If you think you are putting on too much weight, talk with your doctor about it—you may be eating too much of the wrong things.

You'll probably be told by your doctor to consume an additional 300 calories a day *during the second and third trimesters.* (The fetus is so small during the first trimester that most doctors and nutritionists now believe you don't need extra calories then.) If you think about it, 300 calories is not all that much. There are 300 calories in 2 cups of *plain* lowfat yogurt or 220 calories in a baked potato with some vegetarian chili on top. *One* McDonald's sausage and egg biscuit has 520 calories (and 35 grams of fat!). One half cup of Ben and Jerry's butter pecan ice cream has 310 calories (and 25 grams of fat). So you see, it's pretty easy to go over the recommended amount of extra calories pretty fast—and if you are eating junk food, it's especially easy to miss out on nutritious calories.

Pregnancy is a time to think even more carefully than usual about diet—a time to eat healthy, wholesome foods in order to give your baby a nutritional headstart in life—and also to make it easier on yourself when it comes time to get back into shape after childbirth.

5 THE PRE-SYSTEM AND SYSTEM

The System is a blueprint for getting back the tight tone of your midsection and returning to your ideal weight within 6 months after childbirth. Actually some women will accomplish both much faster, especially if they were in good shape before getting pregnant and continued to exercise during pregnancy. Some women may take a bit longer. Obviously, it will also depend on how soon you start exercising after childbirth—some women can start right away, others have to (or simply want to) wait weeks or even months. I'll address this subject in detail a little further down in this chapter, but, ideally, you should start exercising as soon as your doctor or medical caregiver says it's okay. The sooner you're able to start, the sooner you'll be on the beach.

The Four Components of the System

There are four components to this system: ab exercise and stretches, aerobic exercise, diet, and lifestyle hints. All of them are equally important. You can't do just one or two of them.

The ab exercises and stretches are designed to shorten and strengthen the muscles in your midsection. The diet and aerobic exercise components will enable you to lose any excess weight you gained during pregnancy. Some women, especially younger ones who have just had their first child, may find they don't need to lose additional weight—childbirth and breastfeeding pretty much take care of it. If you are one of those women, you should still read the chapter on postpartum aerobic exercise and perform this part of the System. Aerobic exercise has many other health benefits besides keeping your weight down. You should also read chapter eight, Diet and the System, because it is primarily about eating healthfully, which everyone should do.

The Ab Exercises and Stretches

The stretches and exercises for your midsection take approximately 10 to 15 minutes every other day. The 7 stretches do not vary. Five of them are the same ones I gave you to do during pregnancy; in addition, there are 2 new ones. They prepare your abs and lower back for exercise by getting blood to the area and stretching the muscles of the lower back so you're able to move more comfortably. You can also do the stretches again after the exercises to help the muscles recover.

The exercises increase gradually in difficulty and intensity because your ab muscles will get stronger every time you do them. If you are a regular exerciser you will probably know some abdominal exercises, such as sit-ups and leg raises, that are not included in this book. These and certain others place a lot of stress on the lower back and hip flexors, which is a particular problem for women who've just given birth—because these areas become weakened and stressed during pregnancy. So, I've chosen only exercises that place minimum stress on the back and hips—a good idea in any case. You're trying to exercise your abdominals—not your hip flexors.

Despite that limitation, I try to give you as much variety as possible. The same exercises over and over can get boring—which leads to giving up. So as your abdominal tone returns, I add different and more challenging exercises.

Aerobic Exercise

The second component is aerobic conditioning. This is absolutely crucial in helping you lose any excess weight you gained during pregnancy. Aerobic conditioning consists of any activity that raises your heart rate—for instance, walking, jogging, bicycling, swimming, hiking, etc. Raising your heart rate raises your metabolism, so you burn more calories. When you perform an aerobic activity on a regular basis, your body loses fat easier. Countless scientific studies have proven that there are additional health benefits as well—such as reducing cholesterol, and lowering the risk for heart disease and diabetes, improved mood, and higher energy level. Exercising aerobically 3 times a week for 30 minutes per session has proven to be sufficient in providing such benefits to your body. But you may find yourself liking it so much that you end up doing more.

In the system I start you out with 10 minutes of aerobic exercise every other day and build gradually to 30 minutes every other day. It's your choice whether you want to do it on the same days as you do the ab exercises or on alternate days. I find that because large blocks of free uninterrupted time are so rare for new mothers, most women prefer alternate days. That way the System never takes up more than a half an hour a day.

Diet

I call the diet component of the System *The New York Fitness Trainers' Diet Tips*—because it is based on how I and many of my colleagues eat and recommend for their clients. It is *not* a weight-loss diet per se. New mothers, especially those who are breastfeeding, need to approach dieting with caution, lest they find themselves constantly fatigued and unable to cope. Most pregnant women and new mothers are told that nursing mothers should not diet; this is not necessarily true. They simply must follow special guidelines, which I'll give in chapter eight. And, as I said above, some new mothers won't need to lose any weight.

The diet component of the System is a set of guidelines, tools, and hints for eating healthy, nutritious food. As with aerobic exercise, you will benefit from the dietary guidelines even if you don't need to lose weight. It's healthy to eat right—just like your mother told you. If you do, you never will have a problem controlling your weight.

Lifestyle Hint

In the month-by-month calendar of exercises and aerobic activities in chapter seven, I have embedded lifestyle suggestions—things you can do any time, anyplace to help you toward your goal of a trim, sexy midsection. Exercise, good posture, and eating right are not things to do every now and then, when you look in the mirror and decide you're looking out of shape or can't fit into the jeans you bought 6 months ago. They are a way of life, something to keep in the back of your mind always, as you nurse, or play with the children, or fix dinner, or go to your office job.

How Do I Find the Time?

Again and again I hear the lament from new mothers: I have no time. Not only is there a newborn to look after and feed, there is still the rest of the family, and perhaps a job as well. Even women who have always considered fitness an important part of their lives may start to believe they don't have the time or the energy left to work out.

Even though the demands of being a new mother may seem overwhelming, it will not help matters to stop taking care of yourself. Figure out how to beg, borrow, or steal a half an hour a day to tend to your body's needs. If you do, you'll find yourself with more energy rather than less. You'll be in a better mood to deal with a crying baby. And knowing that you are caring for your body and seeing the results, will make you feel better about yourself—the first step in good relationships with others, including your baby.

My new-mother clients have developed several strategies to help find that extra half hour a day for fitness. Here are some of them:

- Include the baby. This should be easy when you perform the ab exercises, because they are designed to be done at home—right next to your baby's crib, if you like. I've even tried to include your baby in the exercises, whenever possible. (Of course, this works better as your baby gets a little older and can see facial expressions, support her own head, and sit up.) Many parents have also figured out how bring the baby along for aerobic workouts (for more on this and precautions, see chapter five).

- Babies, alas, are not always in the mood to be exercise partners, so on those days when they are cranky and unaccommodating, try to do your exercises when they are sleeping.

- Make a deal with your husband or another new mother. He or she watches the baby while you work out and vice versa. This works best right after a feeding, because your baby probably likes to be fed by you (also, if you are breastfeeding, you won't have to express milk, and exercise will be more comfortable for you because your breasts won't be full).

The System Does Most of the Thinking for You— but Not All!

I've designed the System to make it easy for you. As much as possible, I try to tell you exactly what to do each day—in order to take the guesswork and the indecision out of the process. But, of course, there is such wide variation among women—in their fitness profiles and goals, their individual bodies, etc.—that you will have to do some customizing for your personal situation. For most of the exercises, both aerobic and for your midsection, I give a range in the number of repetitions, duration, and difficulty. You have to be honest with yourself and neither do more than you can nor take it too easy. As fitness trainers will tell you over and over, you have to listen to your body—push yourself a bit but not to the point of exhaustion or injury.

How Soon After Childbirth Can I Begin the System?

The answer to this question is highly individual. I have one client, Francesca, who was up and walking within hours of childbirth and on the ski slopes a week later! I am certainly not recommending this for you. She was and is extremely fit and had exceptionally easy childbirths, for which she even refused an epidural. Similarly, when the women fitness trainers I work with have babies I'm always astonished by how fast they are back at the gym. On the other hand, some of my clients tell me that they don't feel up to snuff for weeks, or even months, after giving birth.

You must consult your doctor or medical caregiver about when it's okay to begin exercising. If he or she approves, and you feel up to it, and you haven't had any complications during pregnancy and childbirth, there is no reason you can't begin the system 72 hours after childbirth. (If you had any complications during pregnancy or childbirth, your doctor or medical caregiver will tell you when it's okay to begin. That includes even such common complications as cesarean birth. Because this program focuses on the abdominal area, there is a danger you could pull your stitches open if you begin too soon. However, doctors have become so adept at cesarean birth that you will probably get permission to start a couple of weeks after giving birth.)

As a rule, most of my clients start working out again 4 to 6 weeks after childbirth. This amount of time is for both physical and psychological reasons; the excitement of bringing the baby home, a steady stream of visiting relatives, learning how to care for your first child—will probably occupy what little free time you have at first. However, if there are no health reasons you shouldn't begin, and you find yourself procrastinating for no reason—well, what are you waiting for? If muscles aren't used, they atrophy. You're just going to make it that much harder on yourself when you do decide to start working out again.

Whenever you do begin to exercise, you must do so with caution.

This is especially important if you start sooner rather than later: your body does not return to its prepregnancy condition immediately. It will retain fluids for at least six weeks, and your uterus will take that long to shrink back to its normal size. Both your abdominal wall and your pelvic floor will be in a weakened condition. Your joints and muscles will still be looser than usual. So start back slowly and exercise with care. Watch your balance, especially when you get up from a sitting or recumbent position, or perform aerobic activities, because your center of gravity is now changing even faster and more dramatically than it did during pregnancy. Don't push yourself to the maximum in stretches or otherwise, because your muscles and joints are still more vulnerable than usual to strains and sprains.

Can I (and Should I) Do Anything Until I'm Ready to Begin the System?

Yes, there are exercises you can and should do, even while you are still in bed. You can do them safely even if you've had an episiotomy or cesarean birth. They will make your recovery faster and more complete, and they will prepare you for the more rigorous exercises found in the System.

The Pre-System

First of all, you must do Kegel exercises (see pages 20–21) as soon as possible after childbirth, to prevent wasting of the pelvic floor muscles. Your entire pubic area will feel slack, irritated, swollen, and tender—so your instinct may be not to do anything. However, Kegels will make the area feel better. In addition, if you had an episiotomy, your stitches may itch. Doing Kegels pulls the incision together, rather than apart, and it will increase circulation to the area, which will promote healing.

You should try to do 1 set of 5 contractions every hour you are awake, for a total of 50 to 60 a day. This will prevent common problems of pelvic floor dysfunction later—such as incontinence and decreased sexual response. Recently I was in a café in Mendocino, California, when a women at the next table rather loudly announced, "I don't care what anybody tells you—it's not the same for your husband down there after you've had a baby. It's not as tight!" I just barely resisted the urge to go over and tell her, "Start doing Kegels." (I hope she buys this book.)

There are two very gentle abdominal exercises that any woman can and should do while still in bed after childbirth: abdominal contractions and pelvic tilts. These are actually the first two exercises in the System and can be found on pages 67–69. They can be safely done even if you had a cesarean, because like Kegels, they will pull any incision you had together, instead of apart. These exercises will help shorten the abdominal muscles, restoring them to their prepregnancy length. This is crucial because the muscles must be shortened before they can be strengthened. I recommend doing 1 set of 3 to 5 slow abdominal contractions followed by 1 set of 3 to 5 pelvic tilts, with a short rest between each repetition, every hour in the initial days after childbirth.

Diastasis Recti After Childbirth

After childbirth, you must check again for diastasis recti (see page 22), although you need to wait until the third or fourth day—until that time your whole midsection will be too spongy and loose to feel much of anything. You may safely do Kegels, abdominal contractions, and pelvic tilts until then to start toning the area.

If the gap is greater than 1 inch (about 2 fingers wide), then you must close it by doing the following exercises before you begin the System:

Postpartum Abdominal Contractions for Diastasis Recti

Lie in your bed on your back with your knees bent and your feet flat on the mattress. Proceed as on pages 23–24. Perform 5 repetitions every 2 to 3 hours. Remember to go slowly and always exhale as you bring your chin to your chest. You should begin to feel the gap close within days.

When your abs feel strong enough, and the gap has closed some, try to continue each crunch up a bit, so your shoulders roll a little up off the mattress at the top of each repetition. Don't jerk up! *Roll* your spine up as you contract your abs and pull the two sides of the rectus abdominis together with your hands. If the gap starts to widen again, it means you are doing too much too soon—your exercises are pulling the gap back apart rather than bringing it together, as you should. Go back to performing just head raises for a couple of days—and then try again.

Generally, after doing this exercise diligently for 2 weeks or so, the gap should have returned to the normal one half inch and you may continue with the System in the rest of the book. Remember the important thing is to restore muscle strength and close the gap gradually.

Once You Start the System, Write It Down!

I'm a big believer in keeping track of your own progress. If you can look at a diary and see real improvement, it will encourage you to go forward and accomplish still more. So I'd like you to get a notebook just for your work with the System. Get one with an attractive cover that you enjoy looking at and keep it in a special place, so you always know where it is. Each day write down a sentence or two about what you did—which exercises, how hard they were, how many minutes of aerobic exercise you performed, what your weight is. If you were forced to miss a day, write that in too. That way it will serve as a guilty reminder.

Also write a sentence on how you feel about your body each time. Don't compare yourself to fashion models and movie stars. Every woman is different! Compare yourself to yourself—noting any improvements in your flexibility, your energy level, your mood, your muscle tone, and your self-image. Figure out what you still want to work on.

This way you'll have the proof you're getting fitter, healthier, and more attractive right there in your own words!

6

THE SYSTEM AND AEROBIC CONDITIONING

Why Should I Do Aerobic Exercise in Addition to the System Exercises?

Exercises that cause the muscles of your midsection to contract, like pelvic tilts and crunches, are designed to make your abs strong, tight, and toned. However, they won't look that way if a layer of fat is covering them. Fat is stored in your body mainly between the muscles and the skin—so if you have extra fat, it will hide the definition of your abs.

During childbirth and in the weeks immediately following, you lose a good deal of the weight you gained during pregnancy. But it's possible you'll still hold on to some excess fat. For both reasons of health and appearance, you should lose it. The ab exercises of the System are not designed to accomplish that. You must do it through watching your diet and through aerobic exercise.

What Exactly Is Aerobic Conditioning?

Aerobic means "with oxygen." When you do any sustained physical activity (let's say running or bicycling), your body needs more oxygen. As a result, your lungs and heart work harder. If they are called on regularly to do this, they will adapt, like any muscle, and become more efficient—hence, conditioned.

Aerobic exercise helps you lose fat because it makes you burn more calories. As you might suspect, the longer and harder you perform an aerobic exercise, the more calories you burn.

Can't I Lose Any Excess Weight Through Dieting Alone?

You can lose weight through dieting alone, but it's more difficult. And most nutritionists now believe that it is virtually impossible to maintain weight loss without aerobic exercise and other lifestyle changes. New mothers, especially those who are breastfeeding, should not go on radical weight-loss diets. They must make sure to get the proper nutrients they need. Regular aerobic exercise will raise your metabolism, helping you burn more calories as your muscles utilize the fat and glycogen (simple sugar stored in your muscles) in your body for fuel. At the end of the day your body will break down fat deposits and convert them into glycogen to store in the muscles you depleted, so you're ready to work out again tomorrow. And the process of turning fat into glycogen causes you to burn even more calories, so you win twice—once when you exercise, and once as your body recovers.

Is There Any Way I Can Lose Fat Only from My Midsection?

Unfortunately, it is impossible to "spot reduce," or lose fat from one particular area of the body. Doing abdominal exercises will not help you lose fat from your midsection. When you lose fat, you lose it from your whole body, not from any one area you are working out.

If I Don't Need to Lose Weight Can I Skip the Aerobic Component?

Even if you don't need to lose weight, I still want you to perform aerobic exercise as a vital part of the System. Aerobic exercise has been proven to have many benefits for your appearance and health besides weight loss and maintenance. It can help regulate blood pressure, lower cholesterol, raise your energy level, strengthen your heart, lungs, and immune system, and improve your ability to sleep. If you don't know it already, you'll soon discover that aerobic exercise is addictive. Actually, it is one of the few *good* addictions. Most people feel a mood-elevating "high" when they run or swim or bike. After a couple weeks of regular aerobic exercise, you will feel a big difference in your body, your mood, and your energy level. You'll find yourself looking forward to your aerobic exercise, and your body will miss it if you skip it.

How Soon After Childbirth Can I Start Aerobic Exercise?

The answer to this question is as individual as women themselves are. It depends on many factors, including how fit a woman was before becoming pregnant, how rigorously she continued to exercise during pregnancy, whether she had any complications during pregnancy or childbirth, etc. In general, obstetricians will tell you to wait until your 6-week postpartum checkup to begin any exercise regimen. However, if you are an extremely fit woman who had no complications, you may ask him or her about beginning sooner—anywhere from 1 to 4 weeks after childbirth. I have often see elite athletes who had easy childbirths back running or cycling within a week. A few words of caution for athletic women, however. Start back gradually and don't be compulsive or panicked about being out of shape. Remember, the changes in your body in the weeks immediately after childbirth are far more dramatic and occur faster even than those you experienced during pregnancy. This can cause problems with a shifting center of gravity. You many find yourself losing your balance even in simple actions—such as getting in and out of the shower or getting out of bed. In addition, you are more vulnerable to muscle and joint strains and injuries. You can expect vaginal bleeding to last 2 to 4 weeks after childbirth. However, if your vaginal flow (called "lochia") becomes heavier or redder or starts again after you thought it had stopped, contact your medical caregiver and take it easy on yourself! It may be a sign that you are trying to do too much too soon.

For the same reasons listed above, women who are just beginning fitness programs and those who stopped exercising during pregnancy need to be even more cautious. I generally advise them to wait 6 weeks before starting more strenuous aerobic activity such as running, jogging, or cross-country skiing. And of course they should get their doctor's permission. It goes without saying that if you had any complications during childbirth, you must consult your doctor or medical caregiver for permission before beginning any strenuous exercise.

Is There Anything I Can Do in the Meantime?

Definitely. As soon as you feel able, get out and walk. In the Pre-system and the first four weeks of the System, I recommend this as your aerobic activity, starting with a minimum of 10 minutes per session, 3 times a week. But it would be even better if you walked for 10 minutes every day. Begin slowly, and if weather permits, walk outdoors and get some fresh air. If the weather is lousy, or your neighborhood has too much traffic or other unsafe conditions, go to your local shopping mall. (An especially good time is early in the morning when few shoppers are there. Many people do their aerobic walking in malls, so you'll have company.) Or find another enclosed space. Just getting out once a day for a short walk will go a long way toward preventing you from feeling cooped up with a baby.

Increase the duration of your walk a minute or two a day so eventually you're doing 20 or even 30 minutes. Also gradually start to pick up the pace. You should aim to get yourself up to a brisk walk by week 3 or 4—say, to 3 to 4 miles per hour (a slow walking pace is 2 to 2.5 miles per hour).

Once I'm Ready for More Rigorous Exercise, How Do I Choose an Aerobic Activity?

The key to aerobic exercise is that you enjoy it, and that you do it *regularly*. Some people don't give much thought to which activity they pick—they just do what a friend does or settle on something they think they should do. Then they find that they don't enjoy the activity and stop after a few times. Or they get overly enthusiastic, do too much the first few times, get exhausted, and just abandon the whole thing.

As a new mother you face special challenges. You'll almost certainly find that your energy level is not what it used to be. It's hard to think about going out for a run or even hopping on a stationary bike when you're exhausted. So pick something you enjoy doing: swimming, running, biking, hiking, cross-country skiing, or a low-impact aerobics class—there are a lot of options. Experiment and find something you really like. Also, you might want to consider mixing it up a bit. Some people get bored with the same activity day in and day out. If you're one of those, try jogging one day, using the StairMaster the next, bicycling the next.

Whatever you choose, make sure it's convenient. Having to drive 2 hours to a mountain for your favorite hike is not very realistic for an everyday routine.

Set a reasonable goal you know you will be able to accomplish each time. In the System I recommend you start walking 10 minutes a day, 3 times a week (although women who were exercising regularly before childbirth may be able to start with more). This gradually increases to a more strenuous activity for 30 minutes (or more), 3 times a week. You can do your aerobic conditioning on the same day you do your ab exercises or on alternate days, but the key is regularity.

All Aerobic Exercise Is Not Equal

How many calories you burn performing any aerobic exercise depends largely on how vigorously you do it. However, certain aerobic exercises tend to be more or less rigorous by their very nature. Running will burn more calories than walking or hiking. Swimming, unless you do it very vigorously, tends to burn fewer calories than many other activities. The *Journal of the American Medical Association* did a study of typical exercise machines you find at a gym and came up with the following list of how many calories you would typically burn in an hour:

> treadmill: 700
>
> StairMaster: 627
>
> rowing machine: 606
>
> cross-country ski machine: 595
>
> stationary bike with arm rower: 509
>
> stationary bike without arm rower: 498

Of course you can change the whole picture by upping the intensity for any aerobic exercise. One further point: If you're a runner, you'll burn *more* calories running on a track or a trail than on a treadmill. On the latter you're just picking up your feet while the surface does the moving.

Strategies for Fitting Aerobic Exercise into a New Mother's Schedule

If you have a treadmill or a stationary bike, put it in the next room to the nursery. Instead of taking a nap during one of those all-too-short periods when your baby is sleeping try a little cycling or running.

Or walk somewhere when you would normally drive. Eventually you could find yourself jogging to the bank or the store instead of using the car. That's one way of turning a necessary errand into a little time for yourself.

Finding another new mother or friend to exercise with is also a great idea. You'll tend to be more disciplined about exercising if you've got a date to keep. Turning your aerobic activity into a social activity will make it more fun for you, something you look forward to even more.

Take Your Baby with You

More and more I see new mothers and fathers taking the baby with them for aerobic exercise. I think this is a great idea. Talk about early exposure to good fitness habits!

You have several options when it comes to baby carriers. For walking and gentle hiking, there are front packs and back packs. Front packs are for infants, back packs are for babies at least 3 to 4 months old who can hold their own heads up. For bicyclists there are child trailers and rear child seats (for 1-year-olds and over). *Always put a helmet on yourself and another on your baby for bike rides.* Collisions and spills, even at extremely slow speeds, can be very dangerous. For runners and joggers with babies who are at least 6 months old, there are running strollers with oversize wheels.

Some words of caution are in order here. Don't take your baby out in extreme conditions (heat, rain, cold, etc.) and always dress her properly to protect her from cold, overheating, and sun exposure. Generally dress her warmer than you do yourself—remember you are staying warmer by exercising. Be careful of jogging and jarring movements: Babies are delicate and shaking and bouncing movements can cause serious brain injuries. And be especially careful of falls and collisions. Avoid crowded areas and heavy traffic. Don't exercise to the point of exhaustion, where your focus and attention is compromised.

Get the Proper Equipment

Appropriate athletic footwear in good condition will go a long way toward preventing foot and ankle injuries. You'll also find you need a good sports bra as your breasts will be enlarged and tender—this is a real challenge for runners and joggers, especially. Some women tell me they wear two bras—their nursing bra and their sports bra over it.

How Do I Know If I'm Working Out Intensely Enough? Or Too Hard?

How do you know which intensity to work at—or in other words, how fast to run or how hard to pedal? Once you have fully recovered from childbirth, your first aerobic goal is to get your heart rate up to 65 percent to 85 percent of its maximum rate for 20 minutes 3 times a week. Your maximum heart rate can be estimated by taking the number 220 and subtracting your age. For example, a 30-year-old woman's maximum heart rate would be around 190 beats per minute. Multiply that by .65 to find out what 65 percent of it is, and then by .85 to find out 85 percent. You will find a range of 124 to 162 beats per minute.

After you finish 20 minutes of exercise, take your pulse. Most people know how to do this, but in case you don't: Put your index and/or middle finger at your wrist or on your neck to the side of your throat and count the pulse beats for 15 seconds, then multiply by 4.

An easier way of finding the desired intensity is by using the Rate of Perceived Exertion (RPE) scale, developed by the Swedish physiologist Gunner Borg. It is based on your gut feeling about how hard you are working out.

In the RPE scale, standing still has an RPE of 6 and an all-out sprint an RPE of 20. Here is the scale:

6	No exertion at all (standing still)
7	
	Extremely light
8	
9	Very light
10	
11	Light

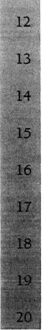

12	
13	Somewhat hard
14	
15	Hard (heavy)
16	
17	Very Hard
18	
19	Extremely Hard
20	Maximal exertion

Throughout the System I refer to the RPE scale to tell you how hard to work out. For the first few weeks in the System, I start you out at 11 and then gradually, over the weeks, I bring you up to the 16 to 17 range. This may sound challenging, but you'll be amazed to see how taking one step at a time takes you to goals you may never have thought possible.

Warning Signs to Stop Exercise and Consult Your Medical Caregiver

A little discomfort is not unusual, especially for those just beginning aerobic routines. But if you experience any unusual pain (especially in your pubic area or lower back), bleeding, dizziness, shortness of breath, nausea, or start feeling faint, or have any other alarming symptoms, stop at once and call your doctor. *Always listen to your body.*

What Should I Do If I Miss an Aerobic Workout?

As I said above, regularity is the key to aerobic conditioning. But every-body misses a workout sooner or later. They're too tired or sick or they just don't have the time on a given day. Some people start missing work-outs—and it's easy to do when you're a new mother—and then just con-clude they don't have the time and give up!

If you have to skip a workout, try to do *something* that day—the 10-minute walk you started with. Then do your regular aerobic workout the next day. Even if you are ridiculously overburdened try for the minimum of 10 minutes a day, 3 times a week. You can *always* afford that much time. Generally it's your attention and focus that are the problem. The holiday season, an important deadline at work, a trip to your parents', a visiting friend—they can all serve as excuses to neglect your aerobic exercise. So you need simply to make it a priority. If you do, you will be richly repaid with good health, a trim appearance, and a self-image that makes you happy.

When you're tired and busy, the hardest part of aerobic exercise is usually thinking about starting, and the next hardest part is actually starting. So don't make excuses about why you can't or won't get going: Just do it. You may feel sluggish at first, but as you start breathing in the invigorating air, and your heart rate rises, and the blood starts pumping through your system, you'll feel a surge of energy you probably didn't even know you had. And the best part will come as you finish. Your body will tingle with good health and newfound vitality!

7 THE EXERCISES AND THE ROUTINES

The following pages contain a 24-week calendar for getting your ab muscles back into shape, plus some guidelines for your aerobic workouts and lifestyle hints. Easy exercises come first—to take into account that your abs are in a weakened condition after being stretched out for nine months and that your lower back is pretty stressed and sensitive. Gradually, as you get stronger, the exercises get more demanding and more varied.

Scheduling the Ab Exercises

The ab exercises are meant to take about 10 to 20 minutes each session, 3 times a week—with a day's rest between each session. So, ideally you should do them Monday–Wednesday–Friday or Tuesday–Thursday–Saturday. I realize that being on such a regular routine is tough for new mothers. So, if your baby has you up all night, or one of your other children is sick, or you are simply feeling exhausted, try to do something that day, even if it's only 3 to 5 minutes worth of the easier ab exercises. Or do your specified routine the next day, which would normally be your day off. (It's okay to do the ab exercises two days in a row *occasionally*.) The key is to maintain some semblance of regularity and somehow to get in your 3 times a week.

The Month-by-Month Calendar

Your workout calendar is divided into 6 months, each month increasing in difficulty, both in the types of ab exercises and in the intensity and duration of the aerobic exercises. The idea, of course, is to move along roughly according to schedule. In addition, the exercises in each month are divided up into two sections, one "Easy" and one "More Challenging." Every month starts with the Easy exercises. Then when they start to feel too comfortable, move on to the More Challenging. Ideally, this should take about 2 weeks.

You should not hesitate to individualize this schedule—both with the number of months and with the 2 sections within the months. Some women may take 3 weeks to move on from the Easy exercises to the More Challenging ones, and 6 or 7 weeks to move on to the next month. That's perfectly okay. Others might go forward more quickly, finding the Easy exercises too easy within a week. If a new routine proves too hard, drop back. However you accomplish it, though, you should make consistent gains in your workouts (meaning more reps, more sets, or less time between sets). As that happens, you will start to see results.

How Do I Really Know When to Move to Each New Step?

You're not out to meet anyone's schedule but your own here. For you a month might be 3 weeks or 6 weeks or 7 weeks, in the System. This 6-month System is only a general guide. Listen to your body carefully and be honest with yourself. Don't cheat yourself by staying at the same level too long; on the other hand, don't be Rambo and charge through the levels. If you do that, you'll probably be performing the exercises incorrectly and too fast. Cheating at your ab exercises is like cheating at solitaire. You're the only one who loses. Always stay focused. If you rush through your session or perform the exercises improperly, you are not going to get the results you want.

My guidelines for aerobic exercise are also very general. The best method for increasing here is to move up a notch—in speed and/or duration—when what you are doing starts to feel too easy. After each aerobic session you should recover pretty easily (meaning your breath and heart rate should return to normal)—within 5 to 10 minutes, say—and you should feel alive and refreshed. If you find yourself feeling totally exhausted afterward, you may be doing too much too soon.

With Ab Exercises, the Most Important Thing Is Correct Form

The most important thing in exercising is correct form. I would rather you did less repetitions with correct form than a lot of repetitions poorly. *Put your mind in the muscle*: The point of each exercise is that you are contracting your ab muscles. Feel that happen. Try to think about how the muscles of the abdomen work from chapter one. Remember that the rectus abdominis pulls the pelvis and the ribs toward each other, and the obliques rotate the trunk. Isolate these specific, desired movements in each exercise and strive to eliminate irrelevant movements, like bobbing your head or swinging your hips or legs around too much.

If you feel the exercises in any given section are too easy for you, check your form, slow down the movements, and make sure you are going through the entire range of motion required before you move on.

Repetitions and Sets

A repetition refers to performing an exercise one time through its full range of motion and returning to the starting position. Each "rep," as most trainers and athletes call them, should be done slowly and in a controlled manner. For each rep, take *at least* 4 full seconds so that you make the ab muscles work—instead of going fast and letting momentum or gravity carry you through the exercise. Remember to return *slowly* to the starting position (but don't rest there). The second part (or negative motion) of any exercise is just as important as the first part. It must be done in a controlled manner, with your abs fighting against gravity. Start the next rep the very instant you hit the starting position. The idea is to keep your abs engaged and contracted throughout the entire "set," which is defined as as a group of reps performed without stopping.

Intensity

Because every woman is different, it is impossible to recommend an exact number of sets and reps for each exercise. So I have included a range of recommended reps and sets as guidelines. You need to customize these. The truth is only you can figure out what you can do and what you need to do. As always, listen to your body. Work until you feel a mild or "good" discomfort, but not until you feel pain, or injure yourself. Be aware of your limits. On the other hand, don't go too easy. Like everything in life, you've got to hit the golden mean. Always aim to build on your strength, adding one or two more repetitions each day or each week.

Equipment

You don't need any! These exercises are designed to be done in your home or just about anywhere you like. You should do them on an exercise mat or a thick carpet for comfort's sake. Wear loose, comfortable clothing and drink plenty of water.

One very popular piece of equipment for ab exercises currently goes by various names. It consists of a metal tubular frame, which goes on the floor to support your neck and arms as you roll up in a "crunch" movement. If you own one of these and enjoy using it, feel free to do so for the appropriate exercises. You'll easily be able to figure out which exercises included in their instruction manual correspond to those we use below. I tend to use this piece of equipment only for my beginner clients to help teach them correct form. As far as the more elaborate ab machines in gyms, such as Nautilus and Cybex, I don't really use them with my clients (or in this book). I believe you can get the same or better results with less risk of back injury by performing exercises that utilize your own body weight. Especially during pregnancy I advise staying away from such machines—they may encourage you to overdo the intensity of your ab workouts.

Stretches

Do all of the following stretches before your first workout. Decide which ones you like and choose at least 3 each time thereafter to do before the ab exercises and before the aerobic workouts. If you have time, do them all. Remember stretching is not a competition. You don't get any gold stars for stretching farther. If you are still recovering from childbirth, you should especially take it easy and not overstretch. The whole point here is to make your body feel *good*, to gently warm your muscles up and prepare them for doing work. When your muscles are warm they are less likely to be pulled or strained by unexpected movements.

Stretching can also be beneficial to help the muscles recover from workouts, so you should try to do them after your workout as well. Stretches are also good to do in the morning, especially if you find yourself waking up feeling stiff.

I. Lower Back Stretch/Strengthen

You may be one of the many women who experience a weakened lower back during and after pregnancy. Here is a good exercise to strengthen it so it will be in balance with your abdominal muscles. Sit in a chair with

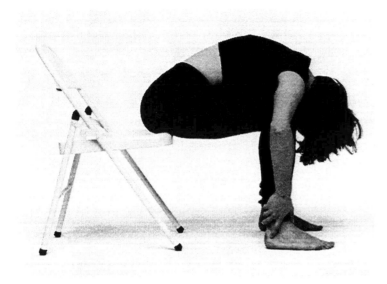

your legs bent at 90 degrees and your feet flat on the floor. Sit up straight—shoulders relaxed, down, and back—then round forward, bringing your head toward your knees, as far as is comfortable, until you feel a slight stretch in your lower back. Try to pull yourself down a little farther by taking hold of your ankles, and exhale as you do so. Suck your abs in at the bottom of the movement. Then, breathing normally, slowly return to the upright position. At the top, arch your back slightly and pull your shoulder blades back down and together. Hold this position for a second, then repeat the exercise. Try to do 2 sets of 10 slow repetitions.

2. "The Cobra" from Yoga

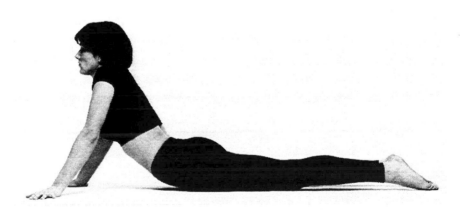

This is a *post*-childbirth stretch, *not* to be done when you are pregnant because your enlarged abdomen will be in the way. Lie on the floor, face down. Put your palms on the floor under your chest. Slowly push your upper body up so your back arches, as far as is comfortable. At the top of the stretch, lift your head up and look at the ceiling. Hold this position for 20 seconds, breathing deeply into your lower back, then go back down slowly to the starting position. Repeat 3–5 times. This is actually a stretch for your abdominals but you will most likely also feel your lower back being taken through its range of motion.

3. The Cat Stretch

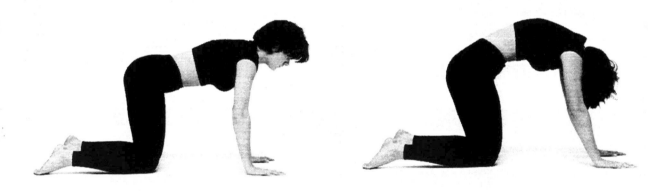

Get down on the floor on your hands and knees. Exhale and round your lower back, pushing the small of your back—not your shoulder blades—up toward the ceiling. Relax your neck and shoulders as your head goes down. Hold the position for 5 seconds, then inhale and slowly go back to the starting position—so that your back is slightly arched.

4. Hip Swing

In the same position as in the Cat Stretch above—on your hands and knees with a slight arch in your lower back—without moving your legs, slowly twist your right hip toward your right shoulder as far as is comfortable, and hold for 2 seconds. Then go back to center, and twist your left hip toward your left shoulder. Make certain you move only your hips in this exercise and not your shoulders. This will stretch the muscles between your hips and your ribs. It also moves your spine from side to side, which should feel good.

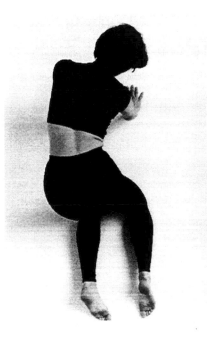

5. Hamstring Stretch

I gave one possibility for stretching the hamstrings in the pregnancy stretching section (see page 28). You can refer to that or try this new one, only to be done after your pregnancy is over. Sit on the floor with your legs out straight and wrap a large towel around your right foot and hold on to both ends of it with your hand or hands. Now lie back and, keeping your right leg straight, raise it up as far as you can. Pull on the towel to get the leg up a bit farther but don't bend the knee. You should feel a mild tension in the hamstring (in the middle of the back of your thigh). Hold that posi-

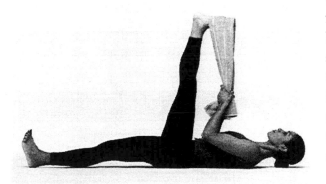

tion for 20 seconds, breathing normally and always keeping your knee straight. Now return to the starting position, and repeat with the other leg. Repeat with each leg. Stretching your hamstrings is extremely important; if they are tight, they can place a tremendous strain on the lower back.

6. "The Pose of the Child," or "The Folded Leaf"

This stretch is also from yoga. Kneel on the floor with your toes pointed back behind you. Lower your butt to your ankles and round your back

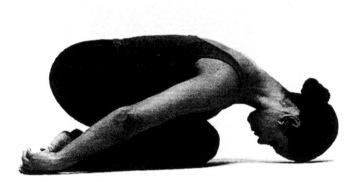

forward so your chest is on your thighs. Reach your hands back toward the bottoms of your feet. Tuck your chin down toward your chest as much as possible. Hold this position for 20–30 seconds, rest, then repeat. This is a great stretch for your lower back and the tailbone area. Many women who have just given birth particularly like this stretch.

7. Hip and Butt Stretch

Lie on the floor on your back, legs out straight. Raise your right leg so the knee bends and comes across your body toward the left shoulder. Grab the right knee with your right hand and the ankle with the left hand. Gently pull both the knee and the ankle across the body, stretching the back and outside of your hip area. Hold that position for 20 seconds then do the other side. Repeat on each side.

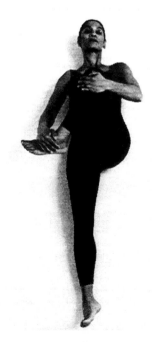

8. Kegel Exercise

I can't remind you often enough to do this exercise. They are not just for pregnancy and the period after childbirth—but for the rest of your life! Do a set of 5–10 repetitions holding each one for 5 seconds. Do them right now as you are reading this.

MONTH 1
EASY

Exercises to be done 3 times a week—with a day of rest between each.

Abdominal Contraction

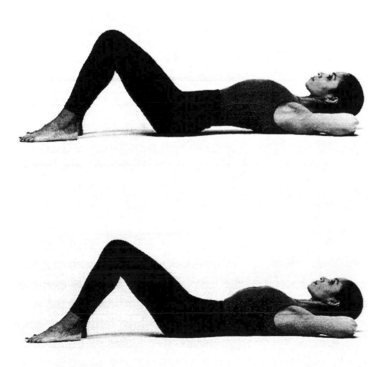

Lie on your back with your knees bent and your feet flat on the floor. Put your hands up behind your head. Now arching your lower back slowly, raise the small of your back off the floor, inhaling gradually as your bellybutton goes up—but keep your shoulder blades and tailbone on the floor. Hold this position for 2 seconds and breathe normally. Then, exhaling gradually, lower the small of your back until there is no curve and it is flat against the floor. You will feel your abdominals contract more and more as you press your lower back into the floor and exhale. This feels good—and you will become aware of your abdominal muscles as they work. Stay in the down position for a 5-second count, then repeat the exercise.

Do 3 sets of 10–15 repetitions with 30 seconds to 1 minute between sets. If your ab muscles feel fatigued by this exercise the first day, then that's enough for you—sometime during the next week you will probably feel strong enough to move on and add the next exercise—pelvic tilts. If you feel you can do more the first day, go on to Pelvic Tilt.

Add a baby: You can sit your baby on your abs facing you for this exercise. The added weight will mean that you'll have to keep your abs tight

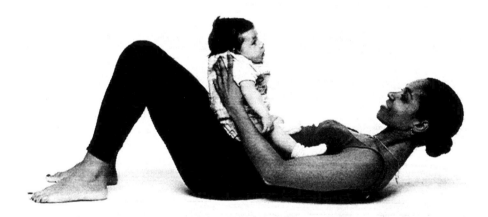

and contracted the whole time, in order to support her. This will increase the difficulty a bit. (Don't use this option during the Pre-System if you had any childbirth complications, such as cesarean birth.)

Pelvic Tilt

Lie on your back with with your knees bent, feet flat on the floor, and hands behind your head. Start by exhaling slowly. Feel your abs tighten as you press your lower back into the floor, as in the previous exercise. Continue exhaling as you slowly roll your hips up and back toward your head, until your tailbone is a half inch or so off the floor. Your lower back should stay on the floor as much as possible—if it comes off you will be using your upper leg muscles, not your abs. (As we saw in chapter one

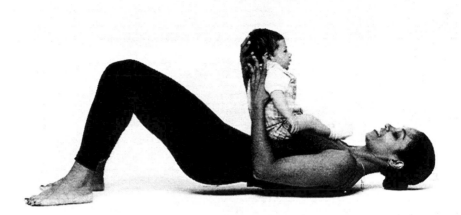

on anatomy, contracting the rectus abdominis brings the pelvis toward the rib cage. This is exactly what you are doing in this exercise. Visualize the muscle working.) Once you reach the top position, inhale slowly and bring your pelvis back down. Keep your lower back pressed into the the floor, do not let it arch up. This keeps the abs working throughout the entire exercise. Once your tailbone touches the floor, repeat the exercise.

Do 3 sets of 10–15 repetitions, with 30 seconds to 1 minute between sets. If you feel fatigued, stop here and call it a day; during the week that follows you will probably feel strong enough to add the next exercise.

Add a baby: Again, sit your baby facing you on your abs for this one. In this exercise you'll actually be lifting the baby's extra weight, so you'll really be putting your baby to work here. If the weight is too heavy, try it without the baby. (This option is *not* to be added in the Pre-System if you had a cesarean or other complication in childbirth.)

Abdominal Crunch

Lie on the floor on your back, feet flat on the floor, knees bent. Place your hands behind your neck to support the weight of your head. Now exhale slowly and press your lower back into the floor. Continue contracting your ab muscles as you roll your spine up so your head and shoulders come up off the floor. (Again, think of the function of your abdominals and visualize them working. As you bring your rib cage toward your pelvis, you will notice that this is the same motion you used in the previous two exercises.) Round your upper back as far as you can

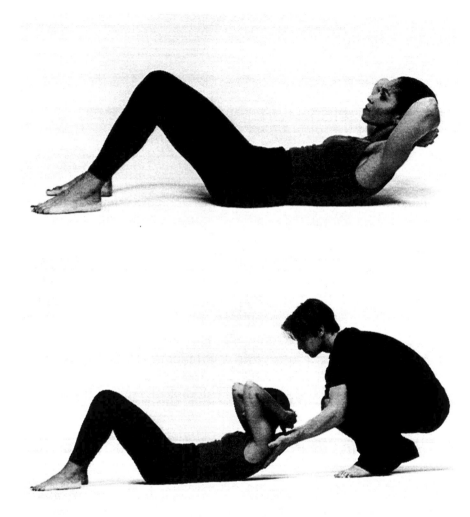

while still keeping your lower back on the floor (continue supporting your neck with your hands).

Try to round up far enough so that your shoulder blades come up off the floor. Always maintain a slow and controlled movement, don't pull hard on the back of your neck or jerk up. Make sure your rectus abdominis is doing the work—feel it working. At first many of my clients can't get their shoulder blades off the floor. If you can't, place a pillow under your shoulders or have a partner assist you by gently lifting your shoulders at the top of the movement. Do 2 sets of 10–15.

Add a baby: Sit your baby facing you, up against your thighs. Support her upper back and neck with your hands if you need to, but try not to tense up your shoulders. Entertain the baby at the top of each rep; for instance, waggle your head a bit and make a funny noise. Your baby doesn't really make this exercise more difficult, but she does stabilize your abs a bit, and she'll probably enjoy helping out.

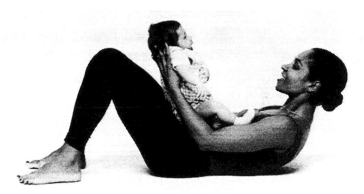

Side Bend

Side bends are mostly for the sides of your midsection (the obliques). Stand up for this one, with your feet shoulder-width apart. Keep your knees bent slightly and let your arms hang at your sides. Continuing to face forward, slowly bend from your waist to the right side, sliding your right hand down the side of your right leg. Visualize your obliques working. Do not move your legs at all. Go down as far as you can comfortably without bending forward. Slowly come back up to a straight standing position. This exercise works the muscles on the opposite side from the direction you bend. Do 2 sets of 15–20 reps to one side and then repeat on the other side.

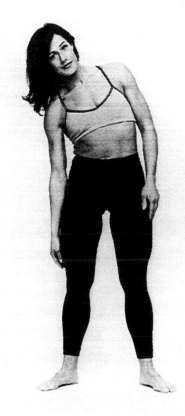

MONTH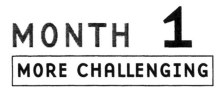

MORE CHALLENGING

Do Abdominal Crunch and Side Bend as described in Month 1 Easy, and Lower Back Stretch (see pages 62–63)

Oblique Crunch

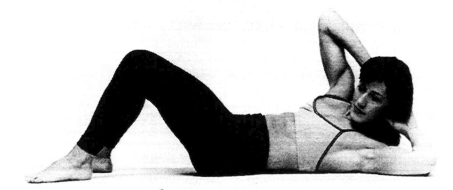

Oblique crunches work all the muscles of the abdominal area, but especially the sides or obliques. Lie on your back with your knees bent and your feet flat on the floor, about 12 inches apart. Place your hands up behind your neck to support your head. Slowly bring your right elbow up and toward your left knee. Go up until your right shoulder blade is off the ground, while your left shoulder blade and left elbow stay on the ground. Don't pull on your neck. Go back down until your right shoulder hits the floor again, but don't let your elbow hit the floor—keep it pointing toward your knee. You should keep your eyes on your knee for the whole set.

You may find it helpful to have a partner assist you by kneeling behind your head, with one hand on your left elbow to stabilize it on the floor, and the other hand under your right shoulder blade to keep it from hitting the floor at the bottom of the movement and to help you go up a little farther at the top.

Do 2 sets of 10–20 of these to the left knee, then the same number to the right knee with the left arm.

Regular Aerobic Activity

It can't be repeated often enough: the key to aerobic workouts is regularity. I know that no new mother gets enough sleep, and you may think that aerobic activity will only make you more tired. Not true. You will have more energy after aerobic exercise. It will also help lift your spirits if you are suffering from the postpartum blues.

For the first 6 weeks after childbirth I do not recommend running, bike riding, or any other activity that will put pressure on your pelvic floor. Your uterus is not back to its regular size yet, and the extra weight is held up by the pelvic floor muscles, which may still be weak. During these weeks stick to walking, swimming, or another low-impact activity that your doctor has approved, to be done at least 3 times a week. Start with 10 minutes of walking at an RPE of 11. You should feel refreshed but not fatigued at the end of the 10 minutes. If you feel you want to walk longer (you may feel it, I swear), then by all means do more. Step up the intensity to 12 if you like, and do another 5 or 10 minutes. Have fun with it. Take a different route each day. Walk with a friend or to a friend's house. Listen to music on a portable CD player (don't do this if you are walking near traffic, however). Anything that will make it more enjoyable will ensure that you keep doing it.

Lifestyle Hint

When you pick up your baby from the crib or bassinet, lift with your legs, not your back. As you lean down, bend your knees, and keep your back flat, with a slight arch in your lower back. (The more rounded your back and shoulders, as in the photo below, the better your chance of pulling a muscle.) Stick your butt back and pick up the baby, keeping her close to your body. Now straighten your knees to rise to a standing position. Also use this motion to pick up

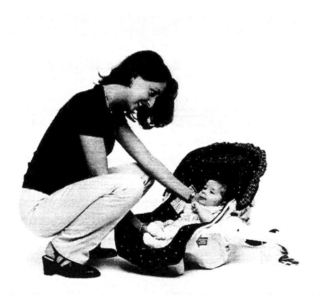

Correct

other things from the floor, like toys. It is a good idea to practice by simply squatting down with the correct motion, as if you were going to pick up something, so it feels natural when you are actually lifting some weight.

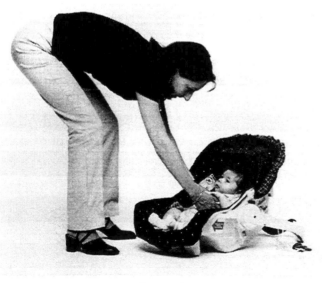

Incorrect

MONTH **2**

EASY

Abdominal Crunch

See the description in Month 1 Easy on page 69. This exercise seems so simple that most people don't realize how effective it can be. It truly isolates the abs. No other muscles are involved, so you can concentrate on your midsection being toned and strengthened. Remember to move from the midsection. Don't just bob your head up and down. Get your shoulder blades off the floor without jerking. Keep the muscles of your entire midsection tight throughout the exercise by not lowering yourself all the way to the floor and not relaxing between repetitions. Don't let your head hit the floor between repetitions, and you'll achieve this.

Visualize what you want your midsection to look like, and feel how with each rep the muscles are getting tighter and stronger. Try to increase the number of repetitions from last month. Aim for 3 sets of 10–20 with good form.

Oblique Crunch with foot on opposite knee

Lie on your back on the floor, left knee bent, foot on the floor, and your right ankle resting on your left knee. Your hands are once again behind your neck to support it. Now, twisting up slowly, bring your left shoulder blade off the floor and your left elbow toward your right knee. Go as far as you can, without moving your knee toward your elbow. Bring the shoulder back toward the

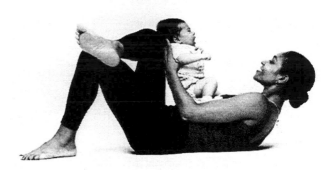

floor (don't let it touch), but keep your elbow pointed at your knee. Do 2 sets of 10–20, then switch to the opposite side and repeat. A common mistake I see people make is to move only from the arm and neck and not enough from the abdominal section, so pay special attention to your form on this one. Twist up from your torso and concentrate on your obliques and rectus abdominis, which are the muscles doing the work here. You can add your baby on this one if she's old enough to sit up: put her facing you, her back supported by your legs and hold her with the nonworking arm.

Side Bend, lying on your side

Lie on the floor on your right side with both legs bent up slightly toward your chest. Extend your bottom arm out on the floor to support yourself; put your top arm behind your neck to support it. Your head should be up off the floor.

Using the left side of your abs, slowly raise your left shoulder so it moves toward your hip. This is a small movement. You will only be

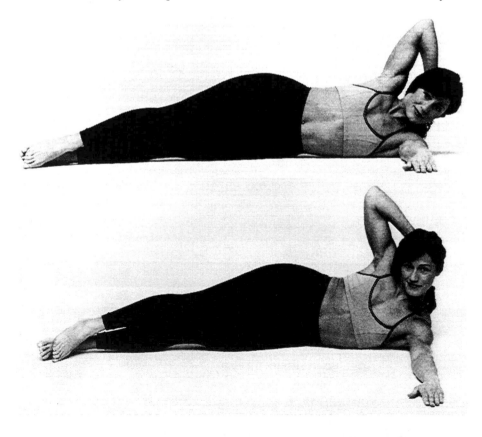

able to move an inch or so. Hold at the top position for a second, then return down slowly. Keep the tension on the muscles between reps by making sure you don't pause at the bottom. Remember the movement is in the side of your abs, so don't just move your neck up and down.

You should feel your sides working within the first 5 repetitions. Try to do 10–15 reps to each side 2 times. Go a little higher, if it seems too easy.

MONTH **2**
MORE CHALLENGING

Simple Reverse Crunch

Reverse crunches are so called because you crunch up from your hips instead of down from your shoulders. Lie on the floor with your knees bent, feet flat on the floor, and your hands under your hips with your palms

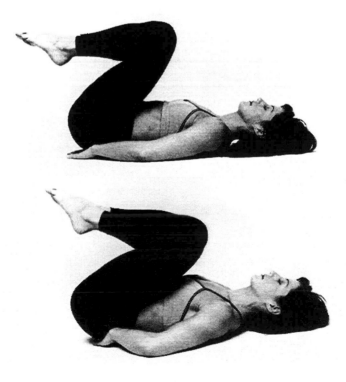

on the floor. Slowly raise your knees and feet up toward the ceiling, causing your hips and tailbone to round up off your hands. Then roll your butt off your hands without using a jerking motion. Lower your hips back down until your tailbone touches the floor (but not your feet). If you are having trouble raising your butt off your hands, still try to do the movement and tighten your abs as much as possible. Try pushing down on the floor with your hands to achieve a greater range of motion. You'll be able to lift your butt eventually.

Your rectus abdominis works in bringing the hips off the floor, not in moving your legs back and forth, so feel it contract, while keeping your legs still. Start with 2 sets of 8–15 reps. As always, increase the number of reps if you need to.

Side Bends, lying on your side with a bent-leg raise

This is similar to the side bends on page 76. Start in the same position: on the floor, on your side, bottom arm extended out on the floor, top hand behind your neck to support it, legs bent up toward your chest. Now tighten your obliques and move your shoulder toward your hip. At

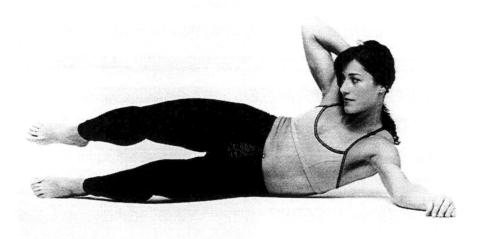

the same time raise your bent top leg as far as you comfortably can. Then lower both your upper body and your leg back to the starting position at the same time. Do 2 sets of 10–20 reps. (One set includes both sides.) Make sure you bend from your torso, not from your neck.

Abdominal Crunch with a pause

Being an expert at crunches by now, you will have no problem adding a pause at the top of each repetition. Count to 2 before coming back down. Your abs will automatically tighten during the pause in order to hold you up. Work hard on these, you won't be disappointed with the results. Do 3 sets of 15–25.

Oblique Crunch with foot on opposite knee

See the description in Month 2 Easy. Do 2 sets of 15–25 reps.

Aerobic Activity

Unless you've been experiencing complications or your doctor says you need to continue to take it easy for any reason, you are probably ready for an aerobic activity a little more demanding than walking. This is where you need to make some decisions. Some of you may prefer running, some may like swimming, or aerobics classes, or bike riding, or hiking, or StairMaster, and so on. Some women like to stick with one thing, others like to mix it up. Whatever you choose, do it for 15 to 20 minutes 3 times each week at the very minimum. Work at an RPE of at least 13. Remember this means you are working at 60 percent of a maximal effort. Again, this is a minimum recommendation. Listen to what your body tells you. Be careful, do what feels good, but don't cheat yourself.

Lifestyle Hint

In order to have a great-looking midsection, you need great posture. If you hunch over and let your shoulders round forward, the muscles of your abdomen will always be relaxed and shortened—i.e., your stomach will stick out. You must stand or sit with your chest up and your shoulder blades back together and down. Your lower back should be slightly arched. Imagine that you are hanging in space from a string attached to the center of your chest.

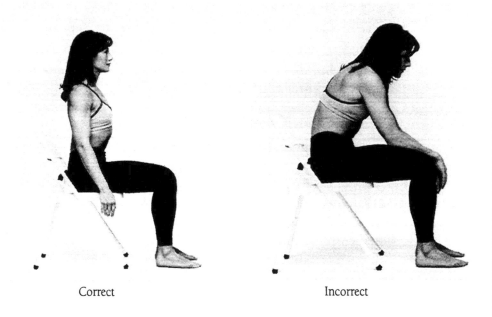

Correct   Incorrect

Great posture takes concentration at first, but soon it becomes second nature. Try to set up Pavlovian signals for yourself. When you see a stop sign remember to sit up straight in the car, or when a television commercial break comes on, pull your shoulder blades back together. An added benefit is that good posture will help prevent injuries and pulled muscles.

Lifestyle Hint

So many things we do in everyday life require us to be rounded and hunched forward—for instance, while you are breastfeeding your baby, you are probably sitting, cradling her with your back and shoulders rounded forward, so your arms can wrap around her. Breastfeeding is one time you shouldn't be

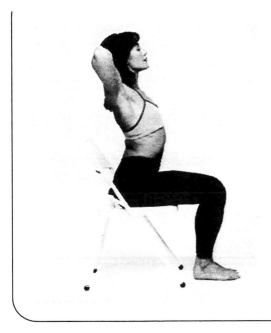

worrying about your posture; your main aim is to stay relaxed. But afterward, it is a good idea to stretch the muscles in your chest and the front of your shoulders so that they don't become tight and pull you into that hunched-over position all the time.

To stretch this area, simply place both hands back behind your head and lift your chest way up in the air while tilting your head back. Arch your back as much as is comfortable and hold that position for 30 seconds. It should feel good when you're done. Do this after every breastfeeding.

Lifestyle Hint

Aerobic exercise dehydrates you, so you should always carry a bottle of water when you run or bike or hike or whatever. This is especially important if you are breastfeeding, because that takes a lot of water out of your system.

At your local sports store you'll be able to find a nifty water bottle for your needs—to mount on the frame of your bike, or to strap around your waist with a tube coming up over your shoulder, so you barely need to use your hands.

I prefer plain water, but most people like something fancier. Don't use soda or 100 percent fruit juice as they are too sugary and will dehydrate you instead of rehydrating you. Sports drinks are okay if you are exercising at high intensity for long periods of time, but they contain a lot of calories. At the level of aerobic exercise you are probably performing here, you'll end up gaining calories if you guzzle down a bottle of a sports drink like Gatorade—and that's probably the opposite of what you're trying to accomplish!

If you *must* have something fancier, add a little fruit juice to your water—at a concentration no greater than 1 part fruit juice to 5 parts water. (But I still wish you would drink just plain water.) Take little sips throughout your aerobic exercise. Drink *before* you feel thirsty. When you're thirsty, you're already dehydrated.

MONTH 3

EASY

Simple Bicycle Movement

Lie on the floor on your back, with your hands under your hips, palms facing down. Lift your legs in the air, until your thighs are perpendicular to the floor, with your knees bent at about a right angle. Push your

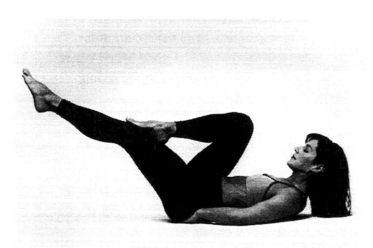

right leg forward and pull your left leg back toward your body at the same time. Without pausing, switch directions and pull your right leg toward your body and push the left leg away. This simulates a bicycle-riding motion if you keep your legs moving continuously. Keep your abs tight throughout. You should feel a mild "burn" in your rectus

abdominis as it fatigues. When pushing one leg forward, be careful not to straighten the knee all the way, as this will put pressure on the lower back. If you are comfortable lifting your head and looking at your legs, do so. This will work your abs a little harder. If your neck gets too tired leave your head on the floor. Do this exercise for 30 seconds, rest for 30 seconds, then do 1 more set. Breathe normally, don't hold your breath.

Crunch with knees bent, feet in the air

Here's a slightly harder variation on the crunches you've been doing. Lie on the floor on your back with your thighs perpendicular to the floor and your lower legs hanging, feet off the floor. Now crunch up slowly as high as you can go. Don't jerk up. It is impossible to go too high, but it is possible to pull on the back of your neck too hard, so be careful. Do

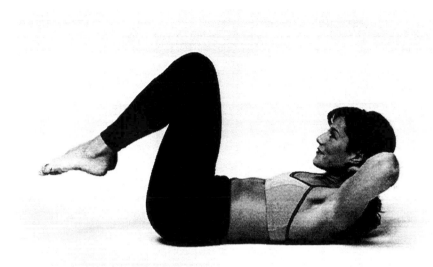

3 sets of 15–25. With your legs in the air your abs have to work just to stabilize your pelvis, which automatically stays still when your feet are on the floor. If you have trouble keeping your legs in the air at first, have a partner assist you by gently stabilizing your legs.

Reverse Crunch

See the description in Month 2 More Challenging (page 77). Lie on your back on the floor with your hands under your hips palms facing down. Slowly raise your bent knees up toward the ceiling and lift your butt up off your hands. Think about rounding your lower back up off the floor and returning slowly until your tailbone, but not your feet, touches the floor. Again, try pushing down on the floor with your hands if you are having trouble lifting your butt. Increase the repetitions to 10–20 for 3 sets. If you do them right, you will feel your abs burning a bit at the end of each set. This means they are working hard, and toning up. If you don't, go back and check your form.

Oblique Crunch with one leg straight in the air

Lie on the floor on your back with your right leg bent and the right foot flat on the floor. Raise the left leg straight up in the air with the knee straight. Put both hands behind your head as you did for the other

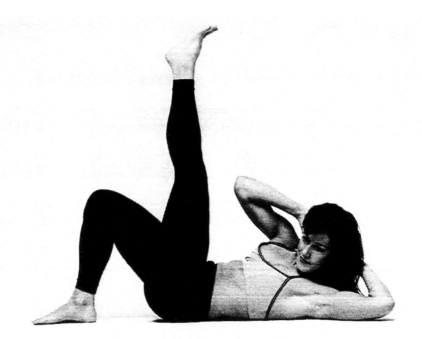

oblique crunches and raise your right elbow toward your left knee that is in the air. Remember to go up so that the right shoulder blade comes off the floor, and don't let the elbow touch the floor when you come down. Keep your eyes on the knee in the air the whole time you are doing the set, and try to keep your hips still. Do 2 sets of 10–15 to each side. Go slow, remember to make it challenging for yourself. It is not the object of any exercise just to get through it, push yourself.

MONTH 3
MORE CHALLENGING

Bicycle Movement with torso twist and a pillow under your head

Lie on your back on the floor, and put a firm pillow under your shoulders. (The pillow makes it easier to hold your shoulders off the floor. As your abs get stronger we'll dispense with the pillow in this exercise.) Put

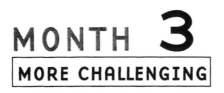

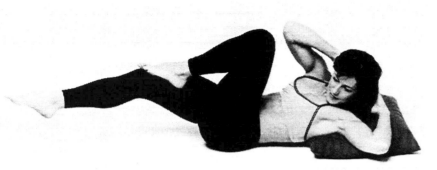

your feet flat on the floor with your knees bent and put your hands behind your neck. Hold your head up so you can look at your knees. Bring the right knee up toward your chest, then the left knee, to begin a bicycle motion with your legs. Don't straighten your leg all the way when you push it forward, this will put pressure on your lower back.

In this exercise you will be moving the upper body also. As you bring your right knee toward your chest, rotate your torso so the left elbow moves toward the right knee. Then as the left knee comes toward you, rotate your torso the other way so the right elbow comes toward the left knee. This is a continuous movement; pick up the rhythm and keep moving from side to side. Do 3 sets of 20 seconds with 20 seconds' rest between each. Make sure you keep your abs tight throughout the exercise.

Crunch with knees bent, feet in the air

See the description in Month 3 Easy (page 82). Do 3 sets of 20–25. Remember to keep your legs perfectly still.

Side Bend, lying on side with straight-leg raise

Lie on the floor on your side with your legs out straight, your bottom arm out in front on the floor to stabilize you, your top hand behind your neck to support it. Now simultaneously raise your top shoulder toward your hip and your top leg about 30 degrees. Make sure you stay on your side throughout the exercise; don't roll back onto your back or forward— your top elbow should be

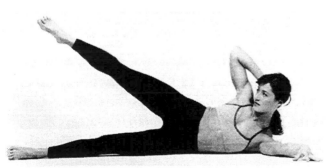

pointing toward the ceiling. Do 3 sets of 10–15 reps to each side, alternating sides.

Reverse Crunch

Do these as you did before (see the description in Month 2 More Challenging, page 77), but try straightening your legs part way, so they are about halfway between being bent at 90 degrees and straight up. As you exhale and push your knees toward the ceiling, feel for the crunch in your abs. Be careful not to let the momentum of your hips carry you through the exercise. Do 3 sets of 12–20.

Aerobic Activity

You should be feeling pretty good by now aerobically. Let's step up the intensity a bit during the next month. Whichever exercise you choose try to work for at least 20 minutes, 3 times each week, at an RPE of 14. If you find yourself not looking forward to doing your aerobic workout each time, pick a new activity. Joining a class or a club is a good strategy to make yourself stick with it. Try a boxing class at the local fitness club, or join a runners' or a cyclists' club. These clubs exist virtually everywhere now, and they usually welcome beginners—so don't be intimidated. An added bonus is meeting people like yourself who want to stay fit.

Remember these recommendations are the bare minimum and you should be working longer at a higher RPE if you feel you can.

Lifestyle Hint

Some of you will be returning to office jobs around this time. Use it as an opportunity for developing healthy fitness-related habits. Every hour, stand up and stretch. Place your hands behind your head and lift your chest way up in the air while tilting your head back. This is good for your posture after you've been hunched over a desk or on the phone for a while. Another strategy: Every time the phone rings, sit up straight, pull your shoulders back and do 5 Kegels.

You can do all this without interrupting whatever you are doing. Also: You can do abdominal contractions sitting right in your chair. No one will be the wiser! As you exhale pull your bellybutton back toward your spine and hold it for 2 to 5 seconds.

Offices are generally pretty dry, so keep a big bottle of water at your desk and drink from it frequently. If you can walk to work, by all means do so. Wear running or cross-training shoes and put your office shoes in a tote bag or backpack.

One big problem in offices is the nearby snackbar or newsstand that carries candy, chips, and cookies. Not to mention the cake, pies, doughnuts, and other food that your well-intentioned coworkers bring in. It's all too easy, when you're hungry or just plain bored, to gobble down unhealthy food in an office. And it's usually impossible to get wholesome food unless you plan for it yourself. So prepare your snacks the night before—it only takes a few minutes. A smart idea is to fill a plastic bag with celery and carrot sticks, or bring in a few pieces of fresh fruit, or some hard-boiled eggs.

It goes without saying that you can pack a healthy lunch for yourself as well. In fact, only you can make a tuna fish (water-packed) sandwich on pita with fresh tomatoes or an egg salad with fresh dill, just the way you like it.

MONTH 4

EASY

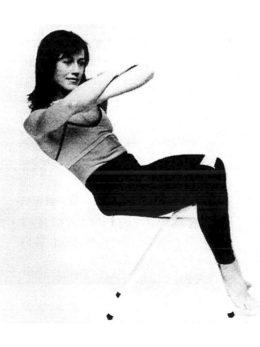

Seated Twist

Sit backward on a sturdy kitchen chair *that won't tip over* (face the back of the chair and grasp the chair with your thighs). Cross your arms over your chest. Lean back just slightly—say, 5 degrees—*again, make sure you will not tip over*. Keep your back straight, don't arch too much or round forward at all. Now twist from side to side rotating from your waist at a medium pace as far as is comfortable. This exercise works the entire abdominal area. Do 2 sets for 20–30 seconds each, with 20 seconds' rest between.

Straight-Leg Reverse Crunch

This is a challenging variation on the reverse crunches you've been doing. Lie on your back with your arms up over your head so you can grab on to a couch, a partner's legs, or something sturdy. With your

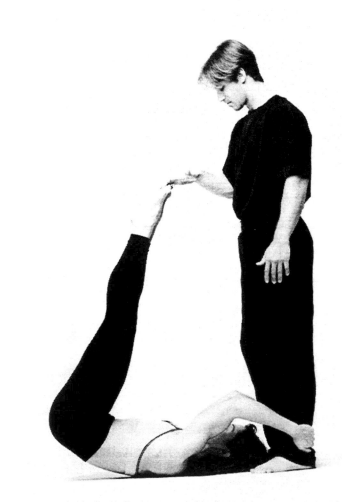

knees as straight as possible, raise your legs so they are back over your chest a bit. Now, raise your hips up about two inches, moving your legs up also. Think about rounding your lower back up so your tailbone comes up no more than two inches off the floor, then slowly lower your hips until your tailbone just touches the floor and repeat. In the down position, be careful to not let your legs go too far forward as this will put stress on your low back. Also, don't keep your legs too far back over your chest. This makes it too easy. This exercise is tricky—so stick with it and think about how the abs work to pull the pelvis toward the rib cage. Try 2 sets of 10–15 repetitions. If you're not able to do these yet, stick with the bent-leg version. (See the description in Month 2 More Challenging, page 77.)

Bicycle Movement with torso twist and a pillow

See the description in Month 3 More Challenging, page 84. Do 3 sets of 20–30 seconds, with 20 seconds' rest between each. Try to move from your torso more than from your neck. It is easy to forget this, so stay focused.

Side Bend, lying on your side with a straight-leg raise

See the description in Month 3 More Challenging, page 85. Do 3 sets of 10–20 on each side. On each rep, pause at the top and count to 2 before lowering to the starting position. When you go up on each repetition, think about the area on your side between your ribs and your hip, which is working.

MONTH 4
MORE CHALLENGING

Greg's Hip Twist

You'll feel this exercise in your entire abdominal area. Lie on your back, hands under your hips, head a bit off the floor. With knees bent, feet off the floor (lower and upper legs should be at about 90 degrees), and moving your legs together, bring both knees toward your left shoulder,

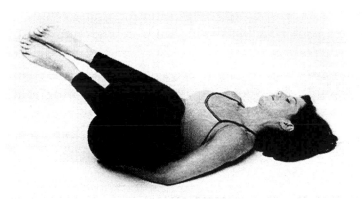

and then lower to starting position. Then, without pausing, bring both knees the other way, toward your right shoulder and then lower them again to the starting position. Keep the movement slow and continuous and try to roll your tailbone up each time without jerking—this is a challenge and you might not be able to do it immediately. Do the best you can and you will get it. Do 2 sets of 10 reps (1 rep includes both sides).

Diamond Leg Crunch

Here is yet another variation of the crunch, which is a bit harder than the last one—because your abs are working without any help from your hip flexors. Lie on your back, put the soles of your feet together, and let your knees fall open—so your legs make a diamond shape. Put your

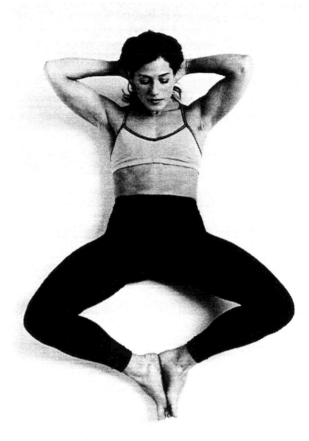

hands behind your neck for support. Now roll up slowly in a crunch as far as you can while keeping your legs still. Do 3 sets of 20.

Bicycle Movement with torso twist, no pillow

Lie on the floor on your back with your hands behind your head. Without the pillow under your shoulders, do the same bicycle movement as in Month 4 Easy, page 89. Try to keep your shoulders, as high off the floor as possible throughout the exercise. Keep moving at a moderate pace. This exercise takes a little coordination, so if you can't get it at first, don't be discouraged. Try to do 3 set of 30 seconds each, with 20 seconds' rest between sets.

Straight-Leg Reverse Crunch

See the description in Month 4 Easy (page 88). These are difficult and it may take some time before you can do them correctly. Keep working on the correct form. Remember to keep your legs as still as possible, don't move them forward and back. Concentrate on rolling up your hips, and keeping everything else still. The abs work very hard when you are raising and lowering only your hips. Do 3 sets of 10–20 reps.

Aerobic Exercise

This month you should be able to increase your workouts to 25 to 30 minutes 3 times each week, working at an RPE of 15. Hopefully, you find it pretty easy to determine your RPE by now.

Athletes like to do a version of aerobic activity called interval training. If you are starting to feel too comfortable in your aerobic workout, try this for a change. In the middle of your aerobic workout, go all-out for 10 seconds, gunning your RPE up to 20. Then drop back to the level you were initially working out at and continue. That may be enough for you, but if you recover quickly, do it again. Build so you can accelerate to peak level a half a dozen times during your 30 minutes. Interval training is an amazing tool for building your endurance, strength, and recovery time. (It also burns more calories.)

Lifestyle Hint

Many elite athletes use a psychological process called "visualization" to help them achieve their goals. For instance, a martial artist visualizes a "round house kick"—that's the classic move you see in martial arts movies where the good guy spins around and kicks the bad guy in the head—at least 10 times before he actually does one; divers do the same with a front 3 1/2 somersault from a 3-meter diving board. Baseball players visualize their swing many times before coming up to bat. Visualization keeps these athletes focused on their goals; it motivates them when they might otherwise be tempted to quit or take it easy.

You can use visualization as well. When you are exercising, keep envisioning how your body works and how you want to look. Imagine a perfect you in a bathing suit on the beach. On those days you feel sluggish and are considering skipping your aerobic workout, go back to that beautiful image and ask yourself, "How much do I really want it?" How much do you want to feel that good about your body? Whenever you are tempted to reach for a pastry or dig into the ice cream, zoom in on your ideal image of yourself. Keep asking yourself, "How much do I want it?" I tell my clients to use that phrase as a mantra; say it every time you are tempted to do something unhealthy.

MONTH 5
EASY

Greg's Hip Twist

If you haven't done this yet then see the description in Month 4 More Challenging (page 89). If you have done this before then increase the range of motion and number of repetitions. Try to do 3 sets of 15–20 reps. Remember to go slow, in a controlled movement; don't let the momentum carry you up, use your ab muscles throughout.

Diamond Leg Crunch

See the description in Month 4 More Challenging (page 90) if you haven't done this yet. If you're an old hand, try to slow down and go a little higher, so your abs work harder. Avoid the temptation to race through an exercise once you get comfortable with it. Do 3 sets of 20–25 reps. If your abs aren't working hard enough, pause at the top and count to 2 before you go down. Remember to exhale on the way up and inhale on the way down.

Abdominal/Reverse Crunches Combined

Lie on your back on the floor, with your hands behind your head, your legs in the air, and your knees bent. Raise your tailbone straight up off the floor, and at the same time crunch your upper body so your elbows

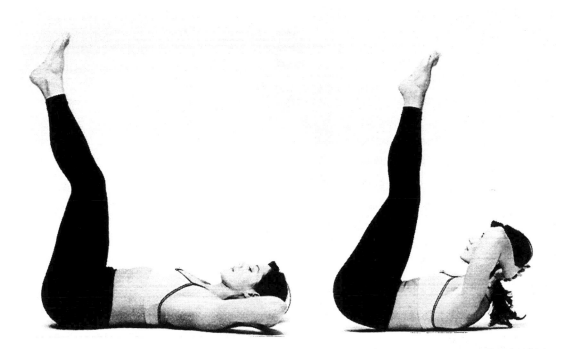

move toward your knees. Then lower your hips all the way down and your upper body down without letting your head hit the floor. When doing the upward motion don't bring your legs too far back over your chest—but you may need to bring them in slightly in order to get your butt off the floor. Moving your legs back and forth involves your hip flexor muscles more than your abdominal muscles, so try to keep your knees right over your bellybutton and move using only your abs. Aim for 3 sets of 10–20.

Straight-Leg Reverse Crunch

See the description in Month 4 Easy (page 88). Aim for 3 sets of 15–25. Concentrate on keeping your legs still. Try adding a 2-second pause at the top before returning your tailbone to the floor. This is a challenge!

MONTH 5

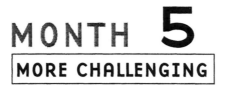

MORE CHALLENGING

Oblique Crunch, one leg straight in air, ankle on knee

Lie on your back on the floor, hands behind your head, right leg straight in the air, and your left ankle on your right knee. Hold your legs as still as possible while you do an oblique crunch, meaning twist your torso so your right elbow moves up toward your left knee. Feel your obliques working as you twist up. Return almost to the starting position, but stop when your shoulder blade touches the floor

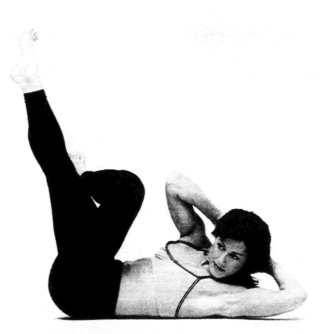

and go up immediately again from there. Do 3 sets of 15–25 reps on each side. Make sure your straight leg is up all the way: If it drops too low, it may put stress your lower back.

Abdominal Crunch, legs straight in the air

Lie on your back with your legs straight up in the air and your hands back behind your head. Do crunches the same as before, keeping your legs still. Try for 3 sets of 30. Add a pause at the top of each repetition if you are not being challenged enough. On the other hand if you cannot

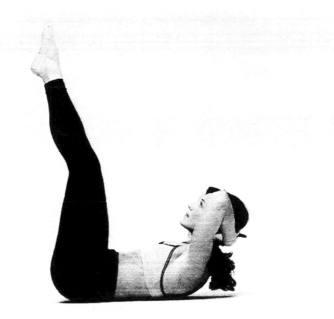

get a good range of motion, try reaching your hands up toward your feet while doing the exercise. I usually make my clients start off with their hands behind their neck, have them do as many as they can, then make them do more with their hands reaching for their feet.

Bicycle Movement with torso twist, no pillow

See the descriptions in Month 4 Easy and More Challenging, (pages 89 & 90). Do 3 sets of 30–45 seconds with no more than 20 seconds' rest between sets.

Abdominal/Reverse Crunches Combined

See the description in Month 5 Easy (page 92). Do 3 sets of 15–25.

Aerobic Activity

If you haven't experimented with interval training yet, give it a try. Your aerobic workouts should be at least 30 minutes long at level 15 or 16. Try putting a 10-second sprint in every 3 or 4 minutes. This is a good goal for anyone. I know not all of you will be up to this, but it's something to aim for even if you can't get it right away. Again make sure you are enjoying your activity, and remember, don't sacrifice your stretching just because your workouts are longer now.

Instead of going out to a restaurant or a movie where you'll be sitting and eating, why not plan a fitness-related entertainment? It'll probably be cheaper, in many cases you'll be able to bring the baby along with you, and you'll feel better afterward. Show off your new aerobic capacity and get in some more endurance work while enjoying activities that are pure fun.

Go hit a few golf balls at a local driving range. Play some night tennis at the local high-school courts (often open to the public after hours). Get some friends together and play basketball or softball—you'll automatically be doing sprints just by the nature of the game. Competitive sports are fun because you get caught up in the moment and forget you're working hard aerobically. Play beach volleyball in the sun or try surfing or wind-surfing or go ice skating or in-line skating. Take a vigorous hike in gorgeous scenery.

As fitness becomes more and more a part of your lifestyle, you'll find yourself searching for any excuse to get out and do something athletic. When you get to this point, I'll guarantee you'll never find yourself bored or depressed.

MONTH 6

PERSONALIZING YOUR AB ROUTINE

Okay, now it's time to start putting together your own ab routines. I've given you plenty of exercises. By this time you know your abs, where their strengths and weaknesses are. You know what your muscles feel like when they are working. You know which exercises work which muscles of the abdominal, which ones you have trouble with, which ones you are good at. A good ab routine is one that you like, because you will keep doing it. But also keep working on those exercises that don't come easily to you at first.

Try to keep your muscles guessing what's next. If they get hit with the same exercises day after day, they stop adapting. You know how to push yourself by now so don't cheat. You're only cheating yourself!

Here are two sample routines of the kind you should start making up.

Routine 1

1. Abdominal Crunch, leg straight in the air, 3 sets of 20–30

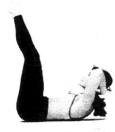

2. Oblique Crunch, one leg straight, ankle on knee, 3 sets of 20–30

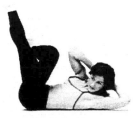

3. Oblique Crunch/Greg's Hip Twist Combined, 3 sets of 15–25

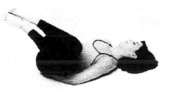

Routine 2

1. Bicycle Movement with torso twist,
    3 sets of 40 seconds, 20-second rest

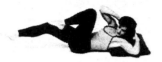

2. Straight-Leg Reverse Crunch,
    3 sets of 15–25

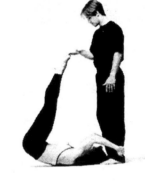

3. Crunches, until you feel a good burn
    in your abs, sets as needed!

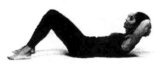

Aerobic Activity

If you have been following the guidelines you should be able to keep a
pretty good pace for at least 30 minutes by now. Working at an RPE of
16 for a half hour will give you an excellent workout. Certainly you can
do more if you are able. If not, then this is your goal.

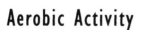

Lifestyle Hint

Sit down and read the journal you've been keeping since you started this
System. Review all the advances you made. Now write out how you feel about

your body at this point. How has it changed since you started 5 months ago? What gains have you made? Perhaps now you can run farther or longer than you ever did; maybe you lost inches off your waist; perhaps you fit into clothes that you haven't worn since before you were pregnant. Think about your self-esteem. How do you feel about your body now as opposed to when you started. Are you better at making time for yourself? How is your mood?

Where do you feel you have room for improvement? Do you still need to lose some weight? Do you need to work on your flexibility? Have you started a particular sport and want to improve your skills? Are you enjoying yourself?

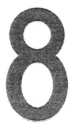 # DIET AND
THE SYSTEM

You can do all the abdominal exercises in the world and develop fabulous, toned muscles in your midsection, but you won't be able to see them—and you still won't fit into your old clothes—if you are overweight. Your sexy new abs will be covered by a layer of unattractive fat. The solution is simple: lose the fat through diet and aerobic exercise! But being a new mother influences how you go about this solution.

As we discussed in chapter four, dieting is not an option during pregnancy. The key then is to make sure you don't eat junk food and gain a lot more weight than your doctor recommends—because you will be stuck with it after childbirth.

After giving birth, you may begin a weight-loss diet after you recover fully. However, if you are breastfeeding, you must lose weight cautiously—always taking into account that you are the major (and perhaps sole) source of your baby's nourishment. A crash diet could hinder your ability to produce milk.

Breastfeeding in itself burns off in the neighborhood of 650 calories a day, so many women assume they will naturally lose weight if they breastfeed. Unfortunately, this is not always the case. The extra demands lactation places on your body will make you hungrier—and you *should* eat more. The problem is that you may find yourself eating so much more, you're not losing any weight at all.

In any case, if you are breastfeeding you can't resort to the usual dieting tactics. You cannot, as you normally might, just cut out most of the fats and/or carbohydrates from your diet—because you don't want to compromise your baby's and your own health by failing to get essential nutrients. You should not resort to diet drugs or liquid or powdered diet formulas—because they can infiltrate your breast milk and harm your baby. You need to eat a balanced, wholesome diet. If you don't, you'll become more and more fatigued as your body drains its store of nutriments to ensure that your breast milk remains nutritious for your baby. In extreme cases, your baby will suffer too.

Eating a balanced diet is always a good idea—*especially* when you want to lose weight, and not just if you are a new mother. But how tempting it is to take shortcuts! They help psychologically, and they're *easy*. Think about it, though—what happens when you go off a fad diet? You put the weight right back on again. Whereas dieting by eating a balanced diet instills good eating habits that will keep the weight off permanently!

How Much Weight Will I Lose as a Result of Childbirth?

Just as women are different in the amount of weight they gain during pregnancy, so are they different in how much they lose during childbirth and in the weeks immediately following. Many of my clients complain to me that they didn't shed as many pounds as they had hoped they would at childbirth. Generally, about 12 to 14 pounds disappears immediately, which includes the weight of the baby and the placenta. In the 2 weeks that follow another 3 or 4 pounds will probably come off, due to loss of fluids. By the sixth week, anything that is left is due to the increased size of your breasts and fat.

Again, it can't be emphasized too strongly that women vary widely (and even different pregnancies with the same woman can be very different with regard to the weight a woman gains and subsequently loses). I've had clients at both extremes. Some have bounced back to their prepregnancy weights within a few weeks of giving birth. In such cases the women were generally lean and in good shape before they got pregnant, continued to exercise throughout their pregnancies (in some cases right up until the day before delivering!), and gained the weight recommended by their doctors, but no more. In other cases, I have had women clients who stopped training with me and otherwise exercising during pregnancy and who put on an extra 20 or 30 pounds.

The Extra Weight Problem After the Second and Third Childbirths

Many women I see have little problem getting back to their prepregnancy weight after the first child. These women are often younger and fitter than those having their second or third child; there isn't the responsibility of additional children, so more time is available for a postpartum fitness routine. It's after the second or third childbirth that I most often hear the complaint, "I lost all but 5 or 10 pounds after I had the baby, and it won't come off—no matter what."

The Psychological Barriers

The months following childbirth can be a tough time to lose excess weight. Caring for a newborn takes most of your time, energy, and focus. The rest of the family may be unusually demanding, as they compete with the new baby for attention. Who has time to think about a complicated diet, count calories or grams of fat, or prepare special diet food different from everyone else's? In addition, most women suffer from some form of postpartum depression, starting a week or two after the baby arrives. You feel let down and depressed, your self-esteem is at a low ebb—the result of your hormone levels returning to normal and the excitement of childbirth subsiding. Many women who come to me to train for the first time at this point are discouraged about their bodies.

As these new moms begin to exercise and tune up their diets, I usually see a dramatic upturn in their self-image and their attitude within weeks. Even if there were no other reason (and there are plenty!), I'd recommend fitness and eating right for the sheer mood-elevating qualities that accompany it.

On the Plus Side

If you are breastfeeding, you automatically burn off around 650 calories a day. That means you'll probably lose weight consuming 1800 to 2200 calories a day instead of the 1200 to 1700 calories generally prescribed by weight-loss diets. You can have much more interesting meals and snacks on 2200 calories a day than you can on 1200!!

How Soon After Childbirth Should I Begin a Diet?

You should wait a minimum of 6 weeks after childbirth before undertaking any weight-loss diet. It takes that long for your uterus to shrink back to its normal size and for your body to lose the fluids accumulated during pregnancy. During those first 6 weeks, you'll have enough on your mind without worrying about your diet.

How Many Calories a Day Should I Be Consuming?

According to the Food and Nutrition Board of the National Academy of Sciences' Institute of Medicine, the recommended daily allowance (RDA) for a woman of child-bearing age is 2200 calories a day. If you are breastfeeding they recommend consuming an extra 500 calories a day, for a total of 2700. (They figure the additional 150 calories of the 650 calories a day it takes to breastfeed will come from fat stores you built up during pregnancy.) However, many women find they don't lose any weight at all if they consume this many calories.

What If I Have 5 to 10 Pounds to Lose and I Am Not Breastfeeding?

If you have only five or ten pounds to lose, you may find it comes off without altering your diet, as you perform the aerobic component of the System. Many people discover that aerobic conditioning is the key to weight control—especially if they cut out junk in their diets: candy, doughnuts, pies, cakes, cookies, fast food, etc.—and alcohol. If you get yourself up to 20 to 30 minutes of aerobic exercise at least 3 times a week, there's a good chance you'll soon drop 3 to 7 pounds without altering your diet. This may be sufficient to help you control your weight.

If you do decide you need to go on a weight-loss diet, I'd recommend a gentle, rather than a radical one. After all, there are a lot of demands on your energy right now—you don't need to be fatigued all the time because you aren't getting enough to eat. Try the New York Fitness Trainer Diet tips at the end of this chapter. If you are counting calories, then reduce your intake to 1700 or 1800 calories a day, rather than dropping down to the 1200 that the more extreme weight-loss diets stipulate.

Aim for losing no more than $1\frac{1}{2}$ pounds a week. I know it feels good to get quick results and drop 5 pounds right off the bat. But, if you do that, it will probably be mostly due to dehydration. Virtually all nutritionists agree that gradual weight loss is better. That way you retrain your body and your appetite, so you are far more likely to *keep* the weight off.

What If I'm Not Breastfeeding and Have a Lot of Weight to Lose—Say, 25 Pounds or More?

Some of my clients swear by the professional weight-loss organizations, such as Weight Watchers. Others, with more serious weight problems, have had success with very low-calorie diets, supervised by their physicians. You might also want to seek out the advice of a registered dietitian, who can customize a diet to your particular needs. To find one in your area look in the yellow pages under Dietitian or Nutritionist or call the American Dietetics Association at 800-877-1600.

Can I Diet Safely If I'm Breastfeeding? How Much Weight Can I Lose?

Contrary to popular myth, you can diet while breastfeeding—but you must be cautious. You must make certain that your diet meets the increased nutritional demands that breastfeeding calls for. It is recommended that you do not attempt to lose more than $4\frac{1}{2}$ pounds a month while breastfeeding—which comes to a little over 1 pound a week.

Many of my clients tell me that while they breastfeed, they hang on to an extra five pounds, which comes off without any effort when they wean the baby. Bear that in mind before panicking about a little extra weight.

How Many Calories a Day Should I Consume If I Want to Lose the Recommended Amount of Weight While I'm Breastfeeding?

The answer to this question is, of course, highly individual. You're going to have to find this out for yourself though experimentation.

Theoretically, you should lose some weight if you consume the RDA of 2700 calories—because it is figured to give you a calorie deficit of 150 calories a day. However, many women find that they don't lose any weight eating this much. You may want to start out at the recommended 2700 calories a day, and see what happens. (If you are underweight, you may actually need to consume more than 2700 calories a day.) Then, if you find you are not losing any weight, start gradually reducing the number of calories. Many of my clients find they lose the right amount—about a pound a week—and still get a balanced diet at around 2100 to 2200 calories a day. You should not go lower than 1800 calories a day while breastfeeding unless your physician recommends otherwise.

Also you should bear in mind that while lactating you do need increased amounts of certain nutrients—especially protein. You will secrete 6 to 11 grams of protein a day in your breast milk, so it is recommended you increase your protein consumption by 12 to 15 grams over the usual RDA for women of childbearing age, which is 50 grams.

Some of the other nutrients you'll need more of are vitamin C (found in citrus fruits, tomatoes, green peppers, strawberries, dark-green leafy vegetables), vitamin A (found in eggs, milk, tomatoes, spinach, carrots, sweet potatoes, apricots, winter squash), vitamin E (found in corn and vegetable oil, flax oil, margarine, butter, wheat germ, nuts, egg yolk), calcium (in dairy products, peas, broccoli, kale, mustard and collard greens), vitamin B_6 (in meat, chicken and turkey, eggs, shellfish, avocados, nuts, whole grains, potatoes, beans, bananas), and folic acid (in beans, oranges, eggs, wheat germ, green leafy vegetables). Don't sacrifice a balanced diet in the interest of losing weight.

The Most Popular Weight-Loss Diets

If you decide to go on a weight-loss diet, you'll find no shortage to choose from. Virtually all of those currently popular are one of two types: the low-fat diet and the low-carbohydrate diet. Remember, though, that the bottom line for any weight-loss is burning more calories than you take in.

The Low-Fat Diet

The low-fat diet is generally recommended by nutritionists. It calls for restricting your intake of dietary fats, which occur in large amounts in butter, cooking oils, fatty meats such as sausage and bacon, whole-milk dairy products, cheese, nuts, mayonnaise, and in many processed foods such as cake, pastry, and candy. The theory behind such diets is that fat is high in calories (9 calories per gram, as opposed to 4 calories per gram for carbohydrates or protein) and that your body uses less calories converting dietary fat into body fat than it would converting protein or carbohydrates into body fat.

Nutritionists recommend that you get no more than 30 percent of your calories from fat. On a low-fat diet, you might reduce that to something closer to 20 percent, which would mean around 450 to 500 calories from fat (or 50 grams—remember a gram of fat has 9 calories, so divide 9 into the number of calories) in a 2200-calorie-a-day diet, or 250 calories from fat (or 26 grams) in a 1200-calorie-a-day diet.

You don't need to be a rocket scientist to go on a low-fat diet. Many people do it by intuition by simply limiting their intake of foods they know to be high in fat. If you want to count calories and grams of fat, my advice would be to get a good calorie/fat gram counter, such as *The Complete Book of Food Counts* by Corrine T. Netzer, and reduce your fat intake as per the formula above. Don't cut out all the fat from your diet though—you do need some. Hunters stranded in the wilderness who eat only excessively lean meat such as rabbit eventually starve to death.

The Low-Carbohydrate/ High-Protein Diet

Controversial among many nutritionists is the low-carbohydrate/high-protein diet. It limits your intake of carbohydrates such as sugar, flour, starches, and fruit, and often calls for increased consumption of meat. The most extreme of these diets virtually ban carbohydrates, while telling you to eat all the fat you want. This may sound appealing, but don't fall for such faddish ideas. If it sounds too good to be true, it probably is. Any weight-loss diet you undertake should be based on a balanced diet.

The theory behind low-carb diets is that when your body is denied carbohydrates—its primary energy source—it turns to your fat stores and "burns" them off for energy. Another theory (disputed by many nutritionists and doctors) is that a certain portion of the population has a hereditary problem metabolizing carbohydrates. For them, supposedly, carbohydrates trigger the overproduction of insulin, which in turn causes their fat cells to store more fat.

Weight-lifters tend to emphasize the high-protein aspect of low-carb/high-protein diets because muscle is made of proteins. It's not unusual for them to consume 200 grams of protein a day or more. (To put this in perspective, there are about 24 grams of protein in 3 ounces of steak.) Nutritionists disapprove of protein consumption higher than twice the RDA (around 50 grams a day for adult women, 60 grams for men), because there is some evidence that it might cause kidney problems later in life. However, several recent studies dispute this finding.

Critics of the low-carb/high-protein diet claim that any initial weight loss is due merely to dehydration—because carbohydrates promote water retention and protein acts as a diuretic.

The most popular of the low-carb/high-protein diets are currently Barry Sears's *The Zone* and Michael and Mary Jane Eades's *Protein Power*. In addition, my friend cookbook editor Fran McCullough has written *The Low-Carb Cookbook* for people on these diets.

Which One Is for Me?

Anecdotal evidence has it that people with only 5 to 10 pounds to lose do better on low-fat diets; those with more weight to lose have better success with low-carb/high-protein. I suspect that the different results that people experience are due largely to psychological factors—or to put it more bluntly, which foods you are likely to overeat. When you have a craving for junk food what do you head for—ice cream or candy? Which foods are you less likely to feel deprived of—fatty, creamy foods or starchy, sugary ones? That's probably the key to figuring out which of these diets you're likely to have more success with.

Remember though: the more faddish and restrictive the diet, the worse it is for your body and the less likely you are to stick to it. (In fact, most nutritionists believe the only reason that fad diets don't do more damage is that people don't stick with them long enough!) Especially if you are breastfeeding, stay away from fad and crash diets.

A Pessimistic View

Every year Americans spend between $30 to 50 *billion* on diet books, special foods, over-the-counter remedies and other tools to lose weight. Recently the editors of the *New England Journal of Medicine* concluded the money was largely wasted because "many people cannot lose much weight no matter how hard they try, and promptly regain whatever they lose." The statistics seem to bear out their gloomy view: among Americans extreme obesity has risen 350 percent over the last 30 years, while almost twice as many middle-aged folks are obese. The incidence of adult-onset diabetes has tripled.

The Low-Fat/Fat-Free Fraud

There is a common misconception that dietary fat and body fat are the same thing. Therefore, the misguided thinking runs, if you simply avoid eating dietary fat, you will not put on weight.

This misconception has been ruthlessly exploited by the food industry in recent years as ever-growing numbers of "fat-free," "low-fat," and "reduced-fat" foods have been rushed onto the supermarket shelves. We are now told we can eat all the reduced-fat cookies and candy we want and remain "guilt-free."

If only it were that simple. As we said above, the bottom line—the *only* line, in fact—to weight loss is to burn more calories than you consume. It doesn't matter how you get those calories—as dietary fats, carbohydrates, or protein—because your body does an excellent job of converting *any* excess calories from any source into body fat. The reason to avoid excess dietary fat is that it is more than twice as caloric per gram than proteins or carbohydrates. But, on the other hand, people tend in general to consume larger amounts of carbs and protein.

If you want to test out the thesis that you'll gain plenty of weight from sources that contain no dietary fat, go ahead and add 1000 calories a day to your diet from fat-free sources. Watch what happens to your weight after a month! You'll be huge!

To show you how misleading the current craze for low- or no-fat foods is, let's look at the two-cookie snack-size package of Fig Newtons. The regular packages have 210 calories: the "fat-free" ones have 200 calories (misleadingly labeled as 100 calories per serving size, a serving size being one cookie). You're saving a big 10 calories by eating the fat-free version. A regular Hershey's 1.55-ounce milk chocolate bar has 230 calories, only 30 calories more.

The same is true of many, if not most, fat-free junk foods. They are still high in calories. The sad truth is that, in most cases, eating it is no different than pigging out on regular junk food, which probably tastes a lot better for the extra few calories. Yet people are happily chowing down all over America, believing they are watching their waistlines. *Don't fall into the trap.* Junk food is junk food, no matter what the sales pitch.

The Problem with Dieting

Virtually anyone can lose weight. The problem is keeping it off. The vast majority of people who diet soon put the weight back on again. If you've ever tried dieting, you're probably familiar with the vicious "cycling" that most people who try to lose weight experience: You go on a diet and shed the pounds. You're happy, you feel good, and you slack off. Then you get heavier and feel bad again, so you go on another diet. Each time you go through the cycle it becomes harder to get the weight off and keep it off.

Recently researchers have discovered that there may be a physiological reason for this pattern. They believe your body has a "setpoint," a weight which it will strive to maintain no matter what. If you diet below your setpoint, the theory goes, your hormones will kick in, slowing your metabolism and making you want to eat more. I don't know if it's going to make you feel better or worse to find out that your hormones are sabotaging you, but this is probably why most diet plans are doomed from the start.

Until the pharmaceutical industry comes up with a way to regulate the hormones that maintain your setpoint (and believe me, they are trying!!), the only way truly to maintain weight loss is to reeducate your body and your mind.

The Solution

Nutritionists all believe that dieting is useless unless it is accompanied by a) aerobic exercise (as I say throughout this book) and b) behavior modification. That means that eating healthy can't be a sometime thing. You have to change your life so that you don't even have to think about eating right and you do it all the time. The only diet that *really* works is not a weight-loss diet, it's a healthy diet.

Write It Down

If there are two things people are never honest about—even with themselves—it's food and sex. I urge my clients with persistent weight problems to keep a food diary for a couple of days—to write down *everything* they eat during a given period, including breath mints and milk in their tea or coffee. In that way they can see exactly where their excess calories are coming from.

This may sound like an arduous task, but if you do it you'll be amazed at what you learn about your eating habits. People are notorious for "forgetting" the cookie they grab out of the package when they give one to the kids or the M&Ms they take out of the candy bowl as they walk by it. I knew of one famous chef who was hugely overweight—so much so that when he traveled by plane, he had to book two first-class seats in order to fit his enormous body. There were actually stores he couldn't shop in because he couldn't fit in the door! He arranged to go on a strict weight-loss diet and was following it to the letter, he believed. Mysteriously, he didn't lose any weight. After his nutritionist followed him around for a day or two, the mystery was solved: The chef was helping himself to so many "tastings" in the kitchen of his restaurant that he wasn't consuming any fewer calories at all.

The first step in correcting a problem is to find out what it is. Most of my clients with weight problems discover their problem is junk food and alcohol (which has 7 calories a gram—only fat has more!). Even if you don't need to lose weight, as a new mother you must eat wholesome, healthy, natural foods—not heavily processed ones full of fat, salt, and sugar, so-called "empty calories," so keeping a food diary will tell you valuable things about your eating habits even if you are thin.

The New York Fitness Trainers' Diet Tips

I encourage my clients to try the diet tips that I and many of my colleagues have adopted. Fitness trainers are a highly motivated bunch when it comes to diet and exercise. We can't let our fitness level or our appearance slip. If we put on excess weight, what kind of example would that be to our clients? Who would want to train with us if we sported spare tires around our middles? We have to set a good example.

Like new mothers, we work long hours and have demanding schedules. I often train clients starting at 6:00 A.M. and go pretty much straight through until 8:00 P.M. I squeeze in my own workouts whenever I can, but I do squeeze them in—always. I can't afford to get sick—because if I don't train clients, I don't get paid. And I can't let myself be low-energy, fatigued, or inattentive. This could be dangerous for my clients.

So I have to eat right. After talking with many of my colleagues, I discovered that many of us adhere to the same dietary principles. Most of us have had training in nutrition; we also follow our instincts—after all, if we're not in touch with our bodies, who is? I am willing to bet that these same principles will work for you.

Step 1

Cut the junk out. No trainer I know eats dessert or candy or other junk food. Neither should you. That means no chocolate, doughnuts, cookies, cupcakes, cake, pie, potato chips, soda, highly sugared breakfast cereals, or ice cream. If I want to have dessert, I eat fruit; if I want a snack, I go for a cup of low-fat yogurt.

There is a school of thought that says it's okay to reward yourself every once in a while with a sweet treat of candy or cake as long as you don't overdo it. I am adamantly against this. First of all, it sets up a bad thought process in which you equate junk with a reward. Pretty soon you start "rewarding" yourself every time you feel bad or good or whatever. So forget about using food as a reward. Reward yourself some other way—say, by taking a glorious hike in a beautiful environment or buying yourself a fantastic new pair of running shoes. If you cut the junk out of your diet completely, you'll soon cut it out of your mind as well. It won't even be an option—and you won't have to deal with temptation.

Every time you feel inclined to reach for the candy bowl or order dessert, ask yourself, "How much do I want a trim, sexy figure?"

Step 2

Avoid alcohol. You probably weren't drinking while you were pregnant, so why start again? Alcohol has a lot of calories—an 8-ounce glass of wine has about 200—and virtually no nutritional value. If you drink a couple glasses of wine with dinner, you'll even be less eager to get up with the baby at night. If you are breastfeeding, you should know that alcohol does pass into your breast milk. If you must drink, limit yourself to two 6-ounce glasses of wine a week (and be sure to drink *after* feeding the baby if you're breastfeeding so you don't get your baby drunk; babies' bodies are much smaller than yours).

Step 3

Watch your fat intake. You should be getting no more than 20 to 30 percent of your calories from fat. (If you need to lose weight, your fat intake should be on the low end of this scale.) Say you determine that you should eat 35 to 40 grams of fat a day. It is surprisingly easy to exceed this amount! *One* tablespoon of butter contains 11 grams of fat and 100 calories. One 8-ounce glass of whole milk contains 8.2 grams of fat and 150 calories. Two tablespoons of any prepared creamy salad dressing (Russian, bleu-cheese, Roquefort) will probably contain at least 15 grams of fat and 150 calories. A McDonald's Big Mac has 28 grams of fat and 530 calories and a McChicken Sandwich has 30 grams of fat and 510 calories!

Frankly, I don't count the number of grams of fat I consume a day, and I suspect that few people bother to religiously count fat grams. Try going with your instincts and common sense. Read the dietary labels on packaged food. Use low-fat dairy products, put jam on your toast instead of butter, and dress your salads with low-fat salad dressings, or substitute salsa or low-fat honey mustard. Forget fried foods. Go for turkey, chicken, fish, or lean beef instead of bacon or sausage. Substitute low-fat yogurt for mayonnaise in your tuna fish salad.

Step 4

Get your carbohydrates from natural, whole foods. Limit your intake of processed carbohydrates, such as bread and pasta. Whenever possible get your carbohydrates through whole grains, whole-grain cereals, fruit, rice, beans, potatoes, corn, and peas, etc.

The basic idea here is to cut down on anything that has flour in it. As Dr. Tarnower, the Scarsdale diet doctor, used to say, "If you want to lose weight, take the bread basket off the meal table." Limit your bread intake—to, say, a slice of whole-grain toast at breakfast and perhaps some whole-wheat pita at lunch. Don't serve rolls with dinner. Cut out pasta altogether unless you love it, in which case have it only once or twice a month.

Many people actually gain weight when they start running because they read about "carbo-loading," a technique used by marathoners and other distance runners, who load up on bread and pasta in order to store enough energy to get them through their physical ordeals. But unless you are covering extreme distances—in excess of 8 miles a day—you are not going to burn off the extra calories you consume by carbo-loading.

Get your carbo calories instead from unrefined foods: rice, potatoes, fresh fruit, a delicious bowl of hot oatmeal in the morning!

Step 5

Eat three meals a day. You are awake and active for too many hours with a new baby to skip meals. If you do, you will probably find yourself so ridiculously hungry that you'll binge and eat twice as much as you would have anyway—so eat three full meals a day.

Step 6

Eat three snacks a day, too. If you're like most new mothers, you'll find that you get hungry in the late morning, in the long stretch of mid-afternoon, and at night before you go to bed, or even in the middle of the night when you're up with the baby. You'll be much better off by planning for these times and having healthy snacks available. Otherwise, you'll find yourself digging into a bag of chocolate chip cookies or a quart of ice cream.

Step 7

Summary: Base your diet on whole grains, fresh fruits and vegetables, low-fat dairy products, fish, poultry, and lean meat.

Recommended Breakfast Foods

low-fat yogurt (1 cup: 150 calories, 13 grams protein, 2.5 grams fat)

oatmeal (1 cup: 145 calories, 6 grams, 2.4 grams) and other whole-grain cereals, without added fat or sugar; beware of granola, which is often loaded with saturated fat fruit (1 banana: 105 calories, 1.2 grams, .6 grams; 1 orange: 65 calories, 1.4 grams, .1 grams; 1 apple: 81 calories .3 grams, .1 grams)

eggs (1 egg: 75 calories, 6.3 grams, 5 grams)

whole-grain bread (1 slice: 60 calories, 3 grams, 1 gram) with jam (1 tablespoon: 50 calories, 0 grams, 0 grams) instead of butter or margarine

Recommended Lunch Foods

tuna, packed in water (1/4 cup: 70 calories, 13 grams, 1 gram) (*not* in oil; use low-fat mayonnaise or yogurt for tuna salad)

sliced turkey breast (3 ounces: 170 calories, 23 grams, 2.5 grams)

roast, grilled, or boiled chicken (3 ounces: 160 calories 22 grams, 8 grams)

soup (avoid cream-based soups such as cream of mushroom or New England clam chowder)

salad (use low-fat dressing or salsa or low-fat honey mustard; avoid cobb, chef's, or caesar salad)

baked potato (220 calories, 4.7 grams, .2 grams) (stuffed with any of these: low-fat cheese or sour cream, broccoli, mushrooms, salsa, vegetarian chili)

whole-grain bread (flour tortilla wrap is a good alternative to high-caloric white-bread rolls or croissants, which are loaded with fat)

hummus (1 ounce: 85 calories, 3.5 grams, 4.5 grams) tabouli and salad, raw vegetables on a pita

cole slaw w/low-fat mayonnaise (3.5 ounces: 80 calories, 1 gram, 5 grams)

baked beans, vegetarian (1/2 cup: 130 calories, 3 grams, 2 grams)

fruit

vegetables

Recommended Snacks

crudités (take carrot and celery sticks with you)

low-fat cottage cheese (1/2 cup: 90 calories, 14 grams, 2.5 grams) (flavor to taste with fruit and/or jam; cookbook writer Martha Shulman uses soy sauce, fresh tomatoes, cucumbers, garlic, and vinegar)

baked potato (bake an extra one when you cook, then reheat the next day for a snack)

hard-boiled eggs topped with caponata (an Italian eggplant appetizer) (1 egg with 2 tablespoons caponata: 105 calories, 6.5 grams, 7 grams)

low-fat milk (8 ounces: 121 calories, 8 grams, 4.7 grams) shake with fruit (for instance, a cup of skim milk or low-fat yogurt blended with a banana or fresh strawberries)

graham crackers (8 pieces: 120 calories, 2 grams, 3 grams) and a glass of low-fat or skim (8 ounces: 86 calories, 8.4 grams, .4 grams) milk

fruit

Recommended Dinner Foods

In the next chapter, I give you some of my clients' and colleagues' favorite easy, fast, healthy recipes to inspire you to delicious, simply prepared food. They are ideal for new mothers.

 DELICIOUS, EASY RECIPES FOR HEALTHY EATING

My new-mother clients are some of the busiest women in the world. Many have full-time jobs in addition to their full-time jobs as mothers. Some of them commute to offices an hour or more each way. And they still have to get dinner on the table—so necessity has made them experts in the art of fast and easy cooking.

Living and/or working in New York City, they do have one enormous advantage when it comes to making interesting meals—easy access to an enormous variety of fresh and ethnic foods. The city is packed with small groceries and fruit and vegetable stands, many of them run by people with roots in other cultures: Latin bodegas, Chinese fish markets, Jewish delis, Korean fruit stalls, Italian butchers, Indian spice stores . . . you name it, we've got it. It was once the case that you could get exotic ingredients only in such large urban centers as New York, but with the advent of the 24-hour mega-supermarket, most ingredients, no matter how unusual, are now available everywhere.

I've asked my new-mother clients and the fitness professionals I work with to give me their favorite healthy recipes to pass on to you. The recipes meet these requirements: they have to be delicious; they have to be low-fat; and they have to avoid the use of pasta and bread. If they are high-protein, all the better, in order to meet a lactating mother's increased demand for additional protein. And they have to be extremely easy to prepare, in order to fit in with a new mother's busy schedule.

Chicken Recipes

Roast and grilled chicken is a staple of the trainers' diet. One half of a breast has 29 grams of protein and only 7.6 grams of fat and 193 calories. Compare this with a hamburger, which has 27 grams of protein, 23.5 grams of fat, and 328 calories.

The way *not* to have chicken is fried. A KFC fried breast has 20 grams of fat and 360 calories. A serving of 6 Chicken McNuggets has 17 grams of fat and 290 calories, not counting the dunking sauce. So don't kid yourself if you are eating any of these. Baking is a good substitute for frying, as you'll see below.

Aunt Cele's Spicy Broiler Chicken

Actually, this hearty chicken recipe is not from a new mother, but from a friend's aunt who once worked for Helena Rubenstein in Paris. When she came back to New York in the 1950s, she served this dish to friends in her Greenwich Village apartment.

Salt and pepper

1 frying chicken, cut up, with skin and fat removed

Lemon juice

Soy sauce

Herbes de Provence (rosemary, thyme, oregano, basil, marjoram—and anything else along these lines that you like, fennel seeds and savory, for instance)

Moderately salt and pepper the chicken and put in a broiling pan. Liberally douse with lemon juice and soy sauce, so there is liquid in the bottom of the pan to keep the chicken moist. Put as much herbes de Provence as you like over the chicken—more sparingly will taste more delicate or you can heap it on for a vivid, rustic taste. (You really *can't* put on too much.) Marinate covered in the refrigerator, for a couple of hours if you have time. Grill or broil in the pan for half an hour, turning a couple of times and basting the chicken with the pan liquid to keep moist. Make sure the chicken is done but not dried out.

Yogurt Chicken

Versions of this come from many clients. You can spice it any way you like—to taste Italian or Indian or Middle Eastern. If you don't like yogurt, try this any way. When used as a marinade, it doesn't taste anything like the raw product.

Chicken, cut up and skinned and trimmed of fat

Low-fat plain yogurt

Lemon juice

Garlic

Spices

Salt and pepper

Marinate chicken in yogurt, lemon juice, mashed-up cloves of garlic to taste, plus any of your favorite spices, such as turmeric, allspice, cardamom, chili powder, cloves, etc. Grill or broil as above. Salt and pepper to taste.

Yogurt "Fried" Chicken (which is really baked)

Here is a good low-fat substitute for the greasy real thing. Prepare as above for Yogurt Chicken. Then roll the marinated chicken parts in bread crumbs, drizzle with olive oil, and bake at 375° F. in the oven for 45 minutes.

Roast Chicken with Whole Lemons

This truly amazing recipe, a favorite of several of my clients, was invented by the great Italian cook Marcella Hazan. The heat of the oven steams the juice out of the lemons, which then bastes the chicken—*with no additional fat*—from the inside out.

Roasting chicken, about 2$\frac{1}{2}$–3 pounds

Salt and freshly ground pepper

2 or 3 whole lemons

Preheat the oven to 350° F. Wash and dry the chicken and trim any excess fat. Rub salt and pepper all over the inside and outside of the chicken with your hands. Take the lemons and make 10–20 little holes in each of them with an ice pick or chopstick or some similar instrument. Put the lemons inside the chicken and truss up the chicken with string or cooking needles. Stick the chicken in a roasting pan, breast side down. After 15 minutes, turn the chicken over so the breast is up. Cook for another 20 minutes, then turn the heat up to 400° F. and cook for 15 minutes more.

Cut up the chicken, put on a platter, and pour the pan juices over it. If you like you can put it on a bed of raw watercress, which is how they serve roast chicken at the famous Parisian bistro L'ami Louis.

Fish and Shellfish

Fish is another terrific high-protein, low-fat food. A 4-ounce size serving of sole has 27.4 grams of protein, 1.7 grams of fat, and 133 calories. It's worth an extra trip to the local fish market to get truly fresh fish. Frozen doesn't really cut it; freezing destroys the taste and texture. Plus the fish market will have a much greater variety to choose from.

The following two recipes are from Fran McCullough's *The Low-Carb Cookbook*. Fran is a good friend and one of the great cookbook editors. Fran struggled with her weight for many years—not surprising, considering how much time she spent around food as part of her job. She tried many diets but none of them worked until she encountered Michael and Mary Jane Eades's *Protein Power*. By following their diet—based on high-protein, low-carbohydrates—Fran has achieved a near-miraculous transformation, losing pounds—and keeping the weight off. (Once again, however, I want to say that I don't recommend such extreme dieting for new mothers, particularly if they are breastfeeding.)

Because Fran found there were no low-carb cookbooks, she wrote one. It is superb, reflecting the many cuisines Fran has encountered as a cookbook editor. Because I suggest a *low-* rather than a *no-*carb diet as well as low-fat, I've chosen 2 fish recipes from Fran's cookbook that are low-fat as well as low-carb.

Tuna with Mint, Garlic, and Soy

Easy, unusual, and versatile—you can either grill this tuna or broil it. The key thing is to salt in half an hour before cooking to bring out the flavor.

Per serving   Protein: 34 grams   Fat: 1.4 grams   Calories: 170

Serves 2

2 tuna steaks

Salt

Olive oil

1 garlic clove, minced

1 tablespoon soy sauce

1 tablespoon chopped mint

Lemon wedges

Half an hour before cooking, rub the tuna steaks lightly with salt and olive oil and let stand. Mix together the garlic, soy, and mint. Just before cooking, rub the seasoning into the steaks and either grill or broil 2 minutes per side—the tuna should be rare. Serve immediately with lemon wedges.

Baked Sea Bass

Per serving   Protein: 26.8 grams   Fat: 9.9 grams   Calories: 380

Serves 4

> 1 whole sea bass

Marinade

> 1 garlic clove, minced
>
> $\frac{1}{2}$ teaspoon salt
>
> Pepper to taste
>
> 2 tablespoons fresh lemon juice
>
> $\frac{1}{2}$ cup olive oil
>
> 2 teaspoons dried oregano

Put the fish on a piece of foil large enough to wrap around it.

Make the marinade: In a small bowl, mash the garlic with the salt and pepper. Add the lemon juice and whisk in the olive oil and oregano. Pour half the marinade over the fish and rub it on both sides. Wrap the foil closely around the fish and put in the refrigerator to season for a couple of hours.

Preheat the oven to 350 degrees. Open the foil, pour the remaining marinade over the fish, and seal the package again. Set the fish package on a baking sheet and bake for 40–50 minutes or until the flesh is opaque when tested with the point of a knife. Remove the foil and serve the fish on a platter, hot or cold or at room temperature.

Shrimp in Mustard Sauce

One of my clients, who has just had her second child, works for a movie studio in New York, where she scouts for literary properties for the movies. Her job was so demanding that she stopped exercising during her second pregnancy and put on a few extra pounds. After she came to me, it only took her a few months to get back to her ideal weight. This easy recipe echoes the flavors of her native Sweden.

Per serving   Protein: 9 grams   Fat: 7 grams   Calories: 120

Serves 4

  2 dozen raw shrimp, shelled, cleaned, washed, and dried

  1 teaspoon caraway seeds

  2 tablespoons Dijon mustard

  Pinch of salt

  Juice of 1 lemon

  Fresh dill, chopped

Sauté the shrimp and caraway seeds in a little vegetable oil for 3–4 minutes. Add the mustard, salt, and lemon juice, and stir well. Cover the pan and cook for 5–6 minutes. Stir in the dill and serve.

Vegetarian Dishes

Some people find the idea of plain steamed vegetables too awful to contemplate. Frankly, I'm one of them. The following recipes are for people like me.

Sautéed Spinach

Wash a bunch of spinach thoroughly. In a skillet sauté a couple of cloves of garlic, peeled and chopped, in a little olive oil. Add the spinach. Cover and let the spinach cook down for a few minutes on medium-low heat. Then take the cover off, turn up the heat to medium, and sauté for 3–4 minutes. A minute or two before it's done throw in some pine nuts and/or raisins.

Carrots

Try adding mint and cumin seeds to steamed carrots. (Mint is also good on fresh peas.)

Green Beans Provençal

In a frying pan, sauté a couple of chopped cloves of garlic in a little olive oil. Add one chopped tomato, salt and pepper, and cook for 5 minutes, until the garlic starts to brown. Add sliced green beans. Cover and simmer for 10 minutes. Garnish with parsley or basil.

Green Beans and Tarragon

Top and tail green beans. Put in a bowl, cover with microwavable wrap, and microwave until crisp yet tender. Toss with vinaigrette made from red-wine or tarragon vinegar, a handful of chopped shallots, and dried or fresh tarragon.

Leeks Vinaigrette

Leeks are often quite expensive at the supermarket. If you garden, you can grow more than you can eat. They are delicious and last well into autumn and early winter when there are few other fresh vegetables in your garden.

Cut off the roots and greens from eight leeks. Slice down the middle to within $\frac{1}{2}$ inch and rinse well under cold running water. Poach in baking dish with a couple of tablespoons of water by covering with clear wrap and microwaving for 20 minutes.

Remove from oven, remove wrap, and immediately pour on the leeks a Dijon mustard vinaigrette. Let marinate at room temperature until you are ready to eat.

Sirniki (cottage-cheese patties)

Per serving (1 patty)   Fat: 1.5 grams   Calories: approx. 50

This unusual recipe was given to me by a Russian client. Actually it's unusual in this country, but in Russia, she tells me, it is one of the most popular lunch dishes. It sounds a little complicated, but after you make it a couple of times, you'll see it's pretty easy. It does take planning ahead, however.

The night before you plan to eat these, put a pound of low-fat cottage cheese in a strainer, and put that into a bowl. Stick a plate on top of the cottage cheese and then put a weight on the plate—such as a rock. Put the whole thing in the refrigerator overnight, during which time most of the water will drain out of the cottage cheese. In the morning mix an egg yolk into the cottage cheese and chill the mixture for an additional hour. Then form into patties—about 2 inches in diameter and an inch thick (you'll end up with 5 or 6). Stick them back in the refrigerator for four hours at least, (the long chilling time is necessary so the patties will hold together). Spray a frying pan with cooking spray (such as Pam), coat the patties lightly with flour, and fry at medium heat. Turn them only once, to avoid having them fall apart. Serve with no-fat sour cream (per tablespoon: 18 calories) and/or jam (per tablespoon: 50 calories).

Soups

Jeff's Garlic Soup

Serves 2

     8 cloves of garlic, peeled

     1 bay leaf

     Herbes de Provence

     1 teaspoon olive oil

     5 whole black pepper corns

     Sea salt to taste

Put the ingredients in a saucepan with 4 cups of water. Simmer for 30 minutes. In each of 2 large soup bowls put a slice of toasted French bread and 1 or 2 poached eggs. Pour the soup through a strainer over the bread and eggs.

Cold Tomato Soup

This soup is from Francesca, one of my fittest clients. It's incredibly easy. Francesca serves it in the summer and she claims guests always ask for the recipe.

Per serving   Fat: 5 grams   Calories: 130

Serves 4

- 4 cups tomato juice

- 1 ripe tomato, chopped

- 1 teaspoon commercial horseradish

- Worcestershire and Tabasco sauce to taste

- 1 teaspoon Dijon mustard

- Fresh dill, chopped

- Salt and pepper to taste

- 4 hard-boiled eggs, chopped

- 2 scallions, minced

- 2 stalks celery, minced

Combine all the ingredients, mix well by hand, chill, and serve.

Dessert

For dessert I eat fresh fruit. If you're trying to lose weight, limit yourself to 2 cups of fresh fruit a day.

Balsamic vinegar on fresh strawberries ($\frac{1}{2}$ cup: 23 calories) sounds weird but the vinegar actually makes the berries taste sweeter. Give it a try.

In winter, when the apples are starting to get mealy, you can bake them. Peel and core 4 apples, then slice them into bite-size pieces (each apple, peeled: 72 calories). Put into a baking dish with $\frac{1}{4}$ inch of apple cider ($\frac{1}{4}$ inch: 35 calories); dot very lightly with butter (1 tablespoon: 100 calories, 11.5 grams fat) and put a *little* brown sugar (1 tablespoon: 46 calories) or maple syrup ($\frac{1}{4}$ cup: 210 calories) on top. Bake at 325 degrees for 30 minutes.

10 THE REST OF YOUR LIFE

Now that you've been introduced to the System, what do you do for the rest of your life? Obviously you have to keep exercising—you can't slack off and hope to maintain the results you've achieved, let alone continue to improve. Hopefully, fitness is now your recreation. By this time you look forward to your fitness sessions so much and enjoy them so thoroughly that it wouldn't even occur to you to stop. It's been my aim to make exercising and eating healthfully a part of your lifestyle, as much as sleeping and caring for your baby.

By this time you've learned quite a bit about your body and how it responds to exercise and proper diet. If you think about it you'll probably discover that you don't need to be coddled—you don't need the System telling you exactly which exercises to do every day and for how long. You've had to customize your ab and aerobic routines to a certain extent from the very beginning—because, as I stated many times, every woman is different. However, in the last weeks of the System I directed you to customize your routines completely.

Now, using the System as a general guideline, you've got to plan your own new System for the next 6 months. The trick is to keep changing things around, to keep surprising and challenging your body. If your routine starts to get too comfortable, you'll get bored. And you'll stop making gains. And you've got to keep making gains: There's no standing still in fitness. You're going either backward or forward!

This is not as bad as it seems; gains can be much more spread out now. For example, add 2 minutes to your aerobic activity every 2 weeks or months, or add 3 repetitions to a set of Oblique Crunches every month. Small increases like this will make sure your body never adapts to the same old routine. Or just change from one aerobic activity to another. The point is that your exercise regimen must be ever-changing. Keep your body guessing what is coming next. Surprise it every so often by doing a routine that's totally different: Pick different exercises, or order your exercises differently.

That all being said, I do want to suggest some basic guidelines.

Aerobic Activity

A bare minimum for aerobic activity at this point should be 30 minutes, 3 times each week. Some of you will want to do more. Most of the working mothers I train do at least this much and perhaps a little more. Women who really get into fitness may find themselves doing up to an hour a day, 5 days a week. Then, if you get to the elite fitness level—by which I mean women who are pursuing sports at the competition level—we might be talking up to two hours a day. At that level there is a possibility of overtraining unless you make special preparations and take special precautions. You have to make even more certain you're getting enough sleep, eating the right foods and enough of them, and training in a balanced way. It's not likely that you are going to find yourself doing 2 hours a day of intense aerobic activity—but if you do, you should get in touch with fitness professionals—a coach or a trainer—or perhaps join a club or a team of like-minded athletes.

Even in the middle range of 45 minutes to 1 hour of activity, you should take off at least 1 or even 2 days every week. This will ensure you don't burn out, or wear your body down, instead of building it stronger. Remember that your body repairs itself while you rest. Don't cheat yourself out of rest. You will need to pay attention to your body to find the happy medium that gets you the results.

Always remember that the key to aerobic activity is regularity. If you find that you've laid off for a period of time, don't try immediately to leap back to the level you were previously doing. You may injure your body that way. A client of mine took up biking one summer and then laid off during the bad weather of winter. The first nice day the next spring she dashed out and did 40 miles, thereby wrecking her knees for about a month. She should have built up slowly to the long distance again.

Ab Exercises

In order to maintain toned ab muscles you must always exercise them specifically. Generally 10 to 15 minutes, 3 days a week, with 48 hours of rest between workouts is plenty—certainly enough to give you the results you want. You never need to do more that 4 different exercises, with 3 or 4 sets of each. Include exercises for your obliques as well as ones that concentrate on the rectus abdominis. And keep changing your routine to avoid boredom and to keep surprising your muscles. If you're still not getting the results you want, don't do more ab exercises. Look to your diet. You may need to lose more body fat in order for your muscles to show.

If you plan on having additional children, you'll be especially glad that you kept up your ab routine. Women often tell me that it seems harder to get back their midsections into shape after each additional pregnancy. This won't be the case for you if you are in shape going into a pregnancy.

Total Body Training

In my introduction, I said that one of the advantages the System offered was that it included no weight training. My reason was that new mothers seldom had the time for a more time-consuming routine, and they needed to use the time available to concentrate on their midsections.

Some of the more fitness-minded women have probably overcome that time problem and used this book in conjunction with a weight-training program. In any case, at some point your baby is going to grow up and you are going to find yourself with more time on your hands. When that happens, I can't encourage you strongly enough to try resistance-training for your total body. Some women have a prejudice against weight-training. They fear the muscles in their arms and legs and elsewhere will grow too big, and they'll start to look like body-builders. In truth, the chances of that happening are pretty slim unless you want it to happen and pursue that goal rigorously.

Most models and actresses do perform some sort of weight-training regimen. A moderate weight-training program will keep all your muscles toned and give you beautifully shaped legs, arms, back, shoulders, and chest. Also, stronger muscles get hurt less and can perform day-to-day tasks more easily. Almost always I see significant improvements in posture; in addition, weight-training gives you stronger bones and helps prevent osteoporosis.

And here's an amazing fact most people don't know. Weight-training raises your metabolism and thereby helps you burn calories—because stronger muscles are more dense and need more calories to sustain them. You don't have to lift all the weight in the gym to get great results: moderate weights will do it.

Hopefully, all that is enough to sell you on the idea of total-body training. When you're ready to take the plunge, consult a professional. Proper technique and a balanced routine are of paramount importance here. You will certainly find people ready to help at your local gym or fitness center.

Keep Writing It Down

Make a list of goals you want to achieve in *the next six months*. Don't view this as the end of the System. But the beginning of a new one that you design yourself. Any really successful person, whether she is a self-made millionaire or a gold-medal-winning athlete, will tell you that a happy person is one who is working toward a goal. Achieving your goal is one of the best feelings in the world.

I have seen people completely change their bodies and their lives through fitness. If you have been following the System, you are well along on the road to becoming one of those people, and I probably don't have to convince you of the benefits at this point. All I can tell you is to keep going. See you at the beach!

Index

About the Author

GREG WAGGONER is one of New York City's preeminent personal trainers. Certified as a Medical Fitness Exercise Specialist by the American Academy of Fitness Professionals, he also has pre- and post-natal training certification from the International Fitness Institute.

DOUG STUMPF is a senior articles editor at *Vanity Fair*. A former book editor, he also edited *The Complete Book of Abs*.